Ocular Accommodation, Convergence, and Fixation Disparity: A Manual of Clinical Analysis

Second Edition

David A. Goss, O.D., Ph.D.

Professor of Optometry and Clinical Consultant, Binocular Vision Services,
Atwater Eye Care Center, Indiana University, School of Optometry, Bloomington

Foreword by
Henry W Hofstetter, O.D., Ph.D.

Rudy Professor Emeritus of Optometry, Indiana University,
School of Optometry, Bloomington

Butterworth-Heinemann

An Imprint of Elsevier

Boston   Oxford   Melbourne   Singapore
Toronto   Munich   New Delhi   Tokyo

Every effort has been made to ensure that the drug dosage schedules within this text are accurate and conform to standards accepted at time of publication. However, as treatment recommendations vary in the light of continuing research and clinical experience, the reader is advised to verify drug dosage schedules herein with information found on product information sheets. This is especially true in cases of new or infrequently used drugs.

 Recognizing the importance of preserving what has been written, Butterworth-Heinemann prints its books on acid-free paper whenever possible.

Library of Congress Cataloging-in-Publication Data

Goss, David A., 1948–
    Ocular accommodation, convergence, and fixation disparity : a manual of clinical analysis / David A. Goss. — 2nd ed.
        p.   cm.
    Includes index.
    ISBN 0-7506-9497-1 (alk. paper)
    1. Eye—Accommodation and refraction.   I. Title.
    [DNLM: 1. Accommodation, Ocular.   2. Vision Disorders—diagnosis.
    3. Eye Movements.   4. Vision Disparity.   WW 109 G6770 1995]
    RE925.G67   1995
    617.7'55—dc20
    DNLM/DLC
    for Library of Congress   95-13935
                                                                                CIP

British Library Cataloguing-in-Publication Data
A catalogue record for this book is available from the British Library.

For information, please contact:
Manager of Special Sales
Butterworth-Heinemann
225 Wildwood Avenue
Woburn, MA 01801-2041
Tel: 781-904-2500
Fax: 781-904-2620
For information on all Butterworth-Heinemann publications available, contact our World Wide Web home page at:
http://www.bh.com

10 9 8 7

Printed in the United States of America

To my dad, Arthur Goss, my best mathematics teacher

Epigraph

Fame is a vapor, popularity is an accident, and money takes wings. The only thing that endures is character.

Horace Greeley

He who is theoretic as well as practical is therefore doubly armed: able not only to prove the propriety of his design but equally so to carry it into execution.

Vitruvius

Contents

Foreword
Preface

1. Introduction   1
2. Plotting of Phorias and Introduction to ACA Ratios and Binocular Vision Syndromes   9
3. Plotting Blur, Break, Recovery, and Amplitude Findings and Completing Graphs   21
4. Effects of Lag of Accommodation and Proximal Convergence on Zone of Clear Single Binocular Vision   34
5. Definitions of Terms   40
6. Sheard's Criterion   47
7. Percival's Criterion   53
8. Morgan's Norms and Clinical Analysis   62
9. Introduction to Fixation Disparity   67
10. Clinical Use of Fixation Disparity   76
11. Prescription Guidelines for the Vergence Disorder Case Types   94
12. Presbyopia   120
13. Nonpresbyopic Accommodative Disorders   135
14. Introduction to Vision Training for Accommodation and Convergence Disorders   150
15. Further Consideration of Accommodation, Convergence, and Their Interactions   164
16. Other Systems of Case Analysis   185
17. Vertical Imbalances   195

Appendix A: Answers to Practice Problems   199
Appendix B: Equipment Sources   217
Index   218

Foreword

The first edition of this manual accomplished something that had been lacking in optometric education for decades. It served as an elementary but comprehensive analytical document dealing with the clinical variables of accommodation and convergence. It represented their relationships on a common matrix popularly called "graphic analysis." The present edition has the same objective but interprets a greater variety of classical concepts represented in several different testing techniques and procedures.

Professor Goss clearly has in mind only an introduction to basic optometric science and theory rather than any dogmatic orientation of clinical philosophy. He has culled the literature for references that contribute to his coverage and that may be consulted by students who wish to become more familiar with the theoretical or experimental rationale of any given procedure. In other words, this continues to be a beginner's text, a manual or workbook for the optometry student who has just started to measure phorias, fusional ranges, amplitudes, etc., on a live subject and needs to know what to do with the numbers he or she has recorded on a data sheet. Having accomplished this, the student can then undertake advanced courses, experimentation, and clinical prescription requiring additional insight into the physiologic functions of vision.

Needless to say, the long-established practitioner, too, may well experience some recycling benefits from a study of the manual if only as a gratifying refresher and perhaps even as a corrective tool for inadvertent or timely omissions in his or her earlier training.

Henry W Hofstetter

Preface

The purposes of this edition remain the same as the purposes of the first edition: to help the student learn basic concepts of clinical evaluation of accommodation and convergence, and to provide the fundamentals for a systematic analysis of nonstrabismic binocular vision problems. Chapters 1 through 7 are mostly unchanged from the first edition. The remaining chapters have been reorganized and contain much new material.

The kind comments of students and instructors encouraged me to undertake this revision. The primary intended audience of this edition, like the previous one, is first- and second-year optometry students. This edition will help them acquire an understanding of potentially confusing concepts and have some confidence in their initial encounters with patients with nonstrabismic binocular vision problems. Mastery of the concepts in this book also will help them be ready for any of the several books available on vision training techniques, advanced aspects of accommodation and vergence, and diagnosis and management of strabismus aimed mainly toward third- and fourth-year optometry students and established practitioners. This book could serve as a review for third and fourth year optometry students. It also might be of some interest to ophthalmology residents or to vision scientists who seek information on clinical evaluation of accommodation and convergence.

Accommodation and vergence disorders are among the most common clinical conditions the optometrist encounters. The consequences of accommodation and vergence problems range from minor nuisance to significant discomfort to interference with optimal school, recreational, or occupational performance. It is essential, therefore, that the optometrist conduct comprehensive testing of accommodation and vergence, and have a systematic approach to the analysis of those test findings.

The framework for this book is a graphical display of accommodation and convergence data. I have found this to be an excellent teaching tool for conveying the sometimes difficult concepts of accommodation and convergence analysis. I also find it to be an excellent way of assessing the pattern and consistency of patient examination findings. Although I advocate the routine plotting of examination findings for that reason, the principles presented in this book can guide the practitioner in the diagnosis and management of accommodation and vergence disorders, whether or not a formal plot of the data is completed.

I thank Bolesław Kędzia for helpful suggestions for revision of the first edition, Dawn Goss and Brad Goss for photographic work, Terri Hahn for secretarial assistance, Jacque Kubley for graphics work, and Optec International for photgraphs of the Mallett units. I also thank Barbara Murphy and Karen Oberheim of Butterworth-Heinemann for their enthusiasm and patience.

David A. Goss, O.D., Ph.D.

1

Introduction

This manual is an introduction to the organization and analysis of clinical optometric data used in the diagnosis and management of accommodation and vergence disorders. To detect and properly diagnose accommodation and vergence disorders it is important to have a comprehensive battery of accommodation and vergence tests as well as a systematic method for the analysis of accommodation and vergence findings.

Two components of such a systematic analysis are (1) the comparison of a patient's test findings to normal or average values and (2) assessment of the overall pattern of the patient's test findings to recognize a case type. For the former, statistical studies have determined normative values for accommodation and vergence tests.[1] For the latter, an x,y coordinate plot of accommodation and vergence test results can help to identify patterns and internal consistency of test findings and to evaluate accommodation and vergence relationships.

Commonly called "graphical analysis," this x,y coordinate plot is a method of graphing clinical accommodation and vergence test findings to determine the zone in which a given individual has clear single binocular vision. Rules of thumb or systems of analysis can then be applied to guide decisions concerning patient management. By itself the graph portrays accommodation and convergence findings and does not necessitate the use of a particular system of data analysis.[2] This manual will consider the rules and guidelines that are most commonly used with graphs and that have been time-tested and shown to be supported by objective data. It also will discuss fixation disparity, which is a useful clinical adjunct to graphical analysis.

Graphical analysis can be used for the vast majority of optometric patients. It cannot be used for uniocular patients or for patients for whom testing of accommodation or convergence is not possible or practical. Graphical analysis can be adapted for strabismic patients as well as for patients with normal binocular vision, and it can be used for preschool children and for those with presbyopia. Hofstetter[3] summarized the applications of graphical analysis:

1. The interrelationships of accommodation and convergence can be evaluated readily.

2. The interdependence of various findings becomes obvious.
3. Prediction of test findings other than those investigated during the examination is possible.
4. Erroneous findings can be detected.
5. Conventional rules for the prescription of lenses and prisms can be easily applied to the graph.
6. In orthoptics, a guide for determining diagnosis, therapy, and prognosis can be provided.
7. In case reports, a large body of data can be pictorially summarized.
8. An effective teaching aid can be provided.

Forms for the graph can be obtained from various optometry schools. Some schools and some private practitioners have incorporated the graph into their examination forms.

Many graphical representations have been used through the years.[4–7] The earliest dates to Donders in the middle of the 19th century.[8] The one most commonly used today, and the one we will consider here, was developed through the pioneering efforts of Glenn Fry and Henry Hofstetter.[2,9–12]

CONSTRUCTION OF THE GRAPH

In a clinical vision examination, stimulus values are measured, not response values; that is, the lens power used for the accommodative stimulus and the prism power used for the convergence stimulus are recorded. Like Donders' graph, the present-day graph (Figure 1.1) has convergence stimulus on the x-axis and stimulus to accommodation on the y-axis. The units Donders used for convergence were degrees and minutes; today we use prism diopters (Δ). For accommodation, Donders used the reciprocal of focal length in inches; today we use diopters (D).

Donders drew a line obliquely across the graph through the points that indicated stimulus to accommodation and convergence stimulus when target distance was varied without change in lens or prism power. We do the same today. This line is called the "demand line" or the "Donders line." Its significance will be discussed later. For now, we will look at how it is derived; we derive it simply by determining the stimulus to accommodation and the convergence stimulus for various target distances.

If we assume that the ametropia is corrected, the stimulus to accommodation in diopters is the reciprocal of the target distance from the spectacle plane in meters. For units other than meters, we can use the following formula:

Stimulus to accommodation in diopters =

$$\frac{\text{Number of units in a meter}}{\text{Measured units from the spectacle plane}}$$

When we calculate the stimulus to accommodation for various selected test distances, we get the results shown in Table 1.1.

Convergence stimulus represents how much the eyes must converge
from parallelism to fixate a given object binocularly. Convergence stimulus in prism diopters (Δ) can be calculated by means of the following
formula:

$$\text{Convergence stimulus (in } \Delta) = \frac{10 \times PD \text{ (in mm)}}{d \text{ (in cm)}}$$

where PD = interpupillary distance and d = distance of the test object
from the base line (the line connecting the centers of rotation of the
two eyes).

We will refer to the distance from the test object to the spectacle plane
as the "test distance." To determine d, we assume that the distance from
the base line to the spectacle plane is 2.7 cm and add that to the test distance. Thus, for a test distance of 40 cm, d equals 42.7 cm. Table 1.2
shows the calculated convergence stimuli for various test distances

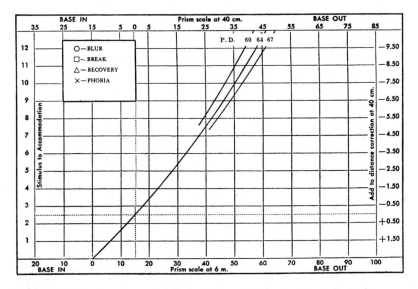

Figure 1.1 The graph currently used for analysis of optometric findings.
The convergence stimulus is on the x-axis and the stimulus to accommodation is on the y-axis. PD, interpupillary distance.

Table 1.1

Stimulus to accommodation for selected test distances. For ease in graphing, the stimulus to accommodation for 6 m often is assumed to be 0.

Test Distance	Stimulus to Accommodation
6 m	0.17D
4 m	0.25D
100 cm	1.00D
50 cm	2.00D
40 cm	2.50D
33.3 cm	3.00D
25 cm	4.00D
20 cm	5.00D
16.7 cm	6.00D
14.3 cm	7.00D
12.5 cm	8.00D
11.1 cm	9.00D
10 cm	10.00D

for one individual with a PD of 60 mm and another with a PD of 64 mm.

One prism diopter of convergence is an eye movement of 1 cm as measured at a distance of 1 m. For fixation of a near-point target the eyes must move in from parallelism of the lines of sight a distance equal to the PD. Therefore, one way to calculate the amount of convergence would be to divide the PD in centimeters by the distance d in meters. The above formula was derived to make use of the most common units for the measurement of PD (mm) and test distance (cm).

To draw in the demand line, we simply plot a point at the stimulus to accommodation and the convergence stimulus for the various test distances for which we made such determinations. Since convergence stimulus is different for different PDs, there is more than one demand line. However, this becomes important only for close test distances. For instance, Table 1.2 shows that the convergence stimuli for these two PDs are only 0.9Δ apart for a 40-cm test distance. This is why demand lines for three different PDs are shown only at the very top of Figure 1.1. For intermediate and further distances, a demand line for only a 64-mm PD is shown, since it is close to the population mean.

By convention, the formula for stimulus to accommodation takes into account the distance of the test object from the spectacle plane, whereas the formula for convergence stimulus uses the distance of the test object from the base line. As a result, the demand line is nonlinear.

Table 1.2
Convergence stimuli (in prism diopters) for various test distances for individuals
with interpupillary distances of 60 mm and 64 mm. Test distance is the distance
from the test object to the spectacle plane. For ease in graphing, the convergence
demand for 6 m often is assumed to be 0.

Test Distance	Convergence Demand 60 mm PD	Convergence Demand 64 mm PD
6 m	1.0	1.1
4 m	1.5	1.6
100 cm	5.8	6.2
50 cm	11.4	12.1
40 cm	14.1	15.0
33.3 cm	16.7	17.8
25 cm	21.7	23.1
20 cm	26.4	28.2
16.7 cm	30.9	33.0
14.3 cm	35.3	37.7
12.5 cm	39.5	42.1
11.1 cm	43.5	46.4
10 cm	47.2	50.4

SCALES ON THE GRAPH

As we have seen, the convergence stimulus is plotted on the x-axis.
A convergence stimulus of 0 represents the situation in which the lines
of sight of the two eyes are parallel to each other, as when they are binocularly fixating an object at infinity. Clinically, distance testing often is at
6 m. We make the assumption that this distance represents optical infinity, so the convergence stimulus (as well as the stimulus to accommodation) for 6 m is assumed to be 0. The base-out values on the x-axis
indicate the number of prism diopters of convergence from parallelism.
Convergence can be stimulated by either moving the target in or adding
base-out prism.

The convergence scale at the top of each graph is there for convenience in plotting near-point findings done at 40 cm from the spectacle
plane since this is the most common testing distance for such findings.
In Table 1.2 the convergence stimulus for 40 cm for a person with a
64-mm PD is approximately 15Δ. Therefore, 0 on the top scale is lined
up with 15 on the bottom scale. A corollary is that if a base-out finding
of 25Δ at 40 cm is obtained, there actually is a convergence of 40Δ from
parallelism.

Stimulus to accommodation can be altered by changing testing distance or lens power. Of course, variations in lens power are considered in relation to the patient's subjective refraction. The scale on the y-axis on the left side of the graph is a dioptric scale for stimulus to accommodation. There also is a scale on the right side of the graph; like the convergence scale at the top of the graph, this scale is designed for convenience in the use of a 40-cm testing distance. Since 40 cm represents a 2.50D stimulus to accommodation, 2.50 on the left-hand scale is at the same place on the y-axis as 0 is on the right-hand scale. Some find it easier to use the top, bottom, and left-hand scales and to ignore the right-hand scale.

TESTS PLOTTED AND SYMBOLS USED

The tests typically plotted in graphical analysis are dissociated phoria**; base-in to blur, break, and recovery**; base-out to blur, break, and recovery**; plus lens to blur*; minus lens to blur*; amplitude of accommodation; and near-point of convergence. Two asterisks indicate tests that usually are done at 6 m and 40 cm, and one asterisk indicates tests usually done at 40 cm; however, any test distance can be used. Some clinicians suggest that tests should be done in the following order: (1) a free-posture test (theoretically no stimulation or inhibition), (2) an inhibitory test, and (3) a stimulatory test. For convergence testing, the phoria would thus precede the base-in, which precedes the base-out. Base-out testing yields a greater fusional aftereffect or vergence adaptation than does base-in testing.[13-15] If the testing order recommended above is applied to accommodation testing, the binocular cross-cylinder would come before the plus-to-blur test, which in turn precedes the minus-to-blur test. Some clinicians do the binocular cross-cylinder test after the plus-to-blur test and before the minus-to-blur test because they feel that the endpoint of the plus-to-blur test is a good starting point for the binocular cross-cylinder test. A first sustained blur is recommended by many clinicians over a blur-out to minimize the effect of depth of focus. However, the graph used in graphical analysis is primarily a means of displaying accommodation and convergence data; therefore, any set of carefully derived findings can be graphed.

By convention, the symbols used in the graph are

phoria: X
blur: circle (○)
break: square (□)
recovery: triangle (△)

These symbols are indicated in the upper left-hand corner of Figure 1.1.

REFERENCES

1. Jackson TW, Goss DA. Variation and correlation of standard clinical phoropter tests of phorias, vergence ranges, and relative accommodation in a sample of school-age children. *J Am Optom Assoc.* 1991;62:540–547.
2. Hofstetter HW. Graphical analysis. In: Schor CM, Ciuffreda KJ, eds. *Vergence Eye Movements: Basic and Clinical Aspects.* Boston, MA: Butterworth-Heinemann; 1983:439–464.
3. Hofstetter HW. The graphical analysis of clinical optometric findings. In: *Transactions of the International Ophthalmic Optical Congress 1961.* London, UK: Lockwood; 1962:456–460.
4. Hofstetter HW. Optometric contributions in accommodation and convergence studies. *Am Optom Assoc J.* 1954;25:431–439.
5. Borish IM. *Clinical Refraction.* 3rd ed. Boston, MA: Butterworth-Heinemann; 1970:875–894.
6. Daum KM, Rutstein RP, Houston G IV, et al. Evaluation of a new criterion of binocularity. *Optom Vis Sci.* 1989;66:218–228.
7. Goss DA. Pratt system of clinical analysis of accommodation and convergence. *Optom Vis Sci.* 1989;66:805–806.
8. Donders FC, Moore WD, trans. *On the Anomalies of Accommodation and Refraction of the Eye.* London, UK: New Sydenham Society; 1864:110–126.
9. Fry GA. Fundamental variables in the relationship between accommodation and convergence. *Optom Weekly.* 1943;34:153–155, 183–185.
10. Hofstetter HW. The zone of clear single binocular vision. *Am J Optom Arch Am Acad Optom.* 1945;22:301–333, 361–384.
11. Fry GA. Basic concepts underlying graphical analysis. In: Schor CM, Ciuffreda KJ, eds. *Vergence Eye Movements: Basic and Clinical Aspects.* Boston, MA: Butterworth-Heinemann; 1983:403–437.
12. Michaels DD. *Visual Optics and Refraction: A Clinical Approach.* 3rd ed. St Louis, MO: Mosby; 1985:380–391.
13. Alpern M. The after effect of lateral duction testing on subsequent phoria measurements. *Am J Optom Arch Am Acad Optom.* 1946;23:442–446.
14. Rosenfield M, Ciuffreda KJ, Ong E, Super S. Vergence adaptation and the order of clinical vergence range testing. *Optom Vis Sci.* 1995; 72:219–223.
15. Goss DA. Effect of test sequence on fusional vergence ranges. *New Eng J Optom.* 1995; 47:39-42.

SUGGESTED READING

Hofstetter HW. Graphical analysis. In: Schor CM, Ciuffreda KJ, eds. *Vergence Eye Movements: Basic and Clinical Aspects.* Boston, MA: Butterworth-Heinemann; 1983:439–464.

PRACTICE PROBLEMS

1. Calculate the stimulus to accommodation for the following testing distances:

   80 cm ___
   75 cm ___
   45 cm ___
   36 cm ___
   30 cm ___
   15 cm ___

2. On the figure below, plot the demand line for an individual with a PD of 70 mm. (Do the necessary calculations.) Where is the most deviation from the demand line for a person with a PD of 64 mm?

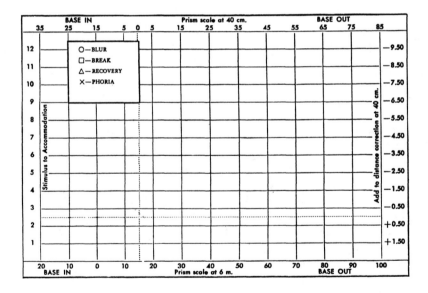

2

Plotting of Phorias and Introduction to ACA Ratios and Binocular Vision Syndromes

As defined in the *Dictionary of Visual Science,* the dissociated phoria is the direction or orientation of one eye, its line of sight, or some other reference axis or meridian, in relation to the other eye, manifested in the absence of an adequate fusion stimulus, and variously specified with reference to parallelism of the lines of sight or with reference to the relative directions assumed by the eyes during binocular fixation of a given object.[1]

In other words, the dissociated phoria indicates the amount by which the lines of sight of the eyes deviate from the condition in which both lines of sight would intersect the object of regard. By definition, the dissociated phoria is measured in the absence of binocular fusion. In phorometric testing the eyes usually are dissociated by a vertical prism.

In exophoria the lines of sight are divergent with respect to the object of regard, and there is a crossed diplopia. During phorometric testing, base-in prism is necessary for vertical alignment.

In esophoria the lines of sight are convergent with respect to the object of regard, and there is an uncrossed diplopia. Base-out prism is required for vertical alignment during phorometric testing.

Most commonly, the phoria is measured in prism diopters (Δ).

PLOTTING PHORIAS

To plot phorias, follow these steps:

1. Find the point on the demand line corresponding to the test distance. Perhaps the easiest way is to determine where the level of accommodative stimulus for that test distance falls on the demand line.
2. If the lenses in place during the phoria test differ from the distance subjective refraction, move straight up one space for each

diopter of minus or straight down one space for each diopter of plus. (The addition of minus lenses over the subjective refraction increases the stimulus to accommodation; the addition of plus lenses reduces it.)

3. Move one space to the right for each 10Δ of esophoria or one space to the left for each 10Δ of exophoria.
4. Mark this point with an X.
5. Connect the X symbols with straight-line segments. The single best-fit line for all the X symbols is called the "phoria line."

Figures 2.1 and 2.2 show examples of phoria plotting. The phoria line should approximate a straight line. If one phoria is way off, the validity of that finding should be doubted. (The use of graphical analysis in the detection of erroneous findings will be discussed later.) In phoria testing, the greatest single source of error is inadequate control of accommodation. To avoid this problem, the examiner should use the smallest letters that the patient can see clearly and should remind the patient continuously to keep the letters clear. Another tactic is to ask the patient to read (aloud) the nonmoving letters forward and backward while the measuring prism is being adjusted.

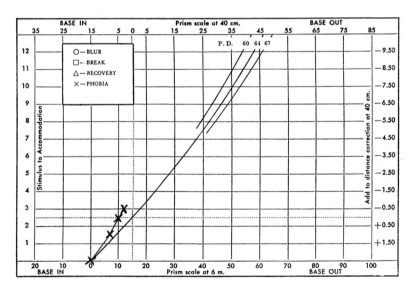

Figure 2.1 As an example of the graphing of phorias and the drawing of the phoria line, the following findings are plotted on the graph:

6 m through subjective refraction: orthophoria
40 cm through subjective refraction: 5Δ exophoria
40 cm through +1.00 over subjective refraction: 8Δ exophoria
33 cm through subjective refraction: 6Δ exophoria

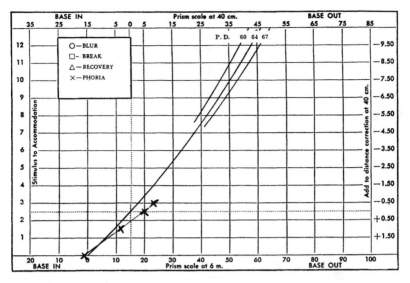

Figure 2.2 Plotting of phorias. This graph was created using data from an individual with the following phorias:

6 m through subjective refraction: 1Δ exophoria
40 cm through subjective refraction: 5Δ esophoria
33 cm through subjective refraction: 6Δ esophoria
40 cm through +1.00 over subjective refraction: 3Δ exophoria

TYPES OF CONVERGENCE AND ACA RATIOS

It is useful to conceive of convergence as being divided into four types: tonic, proximal, accommodative, and fusional.[2,3] Tonic convergence represents the physiologic position of rest. The distance phoria with the subjective refraction in place is taken to be a measure of tonic convergence. Proximal convergence is convergence that occurs because of the psychic awareness of nearness of the target in near-point testing. Accommodative convergence occurs with a change in accommodation as part of the near synkinesis of accommodation, convergence, and pupil constriction.[4,5] Fusional convergence is the convergence that responds to maintain singleness of the object of regard.

In the measurement of a near-point phoria, fusional convergence is eliminated by dissociation and proximal convergence often is assumed to be negligible. (More will be said about this later.) Since the amount of tonic convergence is known from the distance phoria, the amount of convergence that occurs in going from distance to the near-point testing distance is theoretically due to accommodative convergence. Accommodative convergence also can be induced by altering lens power while maintaining the testing distance.

The ratio of accommodative convergence to the change in stimulus to accommodation is known as the stimulus ACA ratio or the clinical ACA ratio. The ACA ratio is the foundation for a large part of clinical decision making.

CALCULATION OF STIMULUS ACA RATIOS

A general formula for the stimulus ACA ratio is

$$\text{Stimulus ACA ratio} = \frac{\text{Accommodative convergence (in } \Delta)}{\text{Change in stimulus to accommodation (in D)}}$$

The formula can be adapted for use with changes in stimulus to accommodation induced by either a change in testing distance or a change in lens power. If two phorias are performed through the subjective refraction, one at distance and one at some near-point distance, the formula becomes

Stimulus ACA ratio =

$$\frac{\text{Convergence demand of near target} - \text{distance phoria} + \text{near phoria}}{\text{Stimulus to accommodation of near target}}$$

The stimulus ACA ratio determined with this formula is sometimes called the "calculated ACA ratio."

In emmetropia or corrected ametropia, the convergence demand and the stimulus to accommodation of the distance target are assumed to be 0. An esophoria is a plus value in the formula, since it represents a convergent posture in relation to the object of regard; an exophoria is a minus value in the formula.

Let's look at an example with this formula. A person with a 64-mm PD has a phoria at 6 m of 1Δ esophoria and a phoria at 40 cm of 4Δ exophoria. Both phorias are taken through the distance subjective refraction. What is the stimulus ACA ratio?

$$\text{Stimulus ACA ratio} = \frac{15 - 1 + (-4)}{2.5} = \frac{10\Delta}{2.5D} = 4\Delta/D$$

The stimulus ACA ratio also can be determined by two phorias taken at the same distance but with different lenses using the following formula:

Stimulus ACA ratio =

$$\frac{\text{Phoria \#1} - \text{phoria \#2}}{\text{Stimulus to accommodation \#1} - \text{stimulus to accommodation \#2}}$$

If a patient has a 40-cm phoria of 3Δ esophoria through −1.00 over the subjective and a 40-cm phoria of 2Δ exophoria through +1.00 over the subjective, the stimulus ACA ratio is calculated as follows:

$$\text{Stimulus ACA ratio} = \frac{3 - (-2)}{3.5 - 1.50} = \frac{5\Delta}{2D} = 2.5\Delta/D$$

The same formula can be used with the gradient test to determine the stimulus ACA ratio. In the gradient test, usually two phorias are performed at 40 cm, one through the subjective refraction and one through +1.00 over the subjective refraction. For example, if the phorias are 3Δ exophoria and 9Δ exophoria, respectively, the stimulus ACA ratio will be

$$\text{Stimulus ACA ratio} = \frac{-3 - (-9)}{1} = 6\Delta/D$$

Stimulus ACA ratios also can be estimated from the graph. Since convergence is on the x-axis and stimulus to accommodation is on the y-axis, the stimulus ACA ratio is the inverse of the slope of the phoria line. If the phoria line is parallel to the demand line, the ratio is 6Δ/D. (This is strictly true only for persons with 64-mm PDs, but it is a good approximation for all PDs close to 64.) A simple example of a stimulus ACA ratio of 6 is given in Figure 2.3. If the phoria line is tipped more toward the abscissa (lesser slope), the ratio is greater than 6; if it is tipped less (greater slope), the ratio is less than 6.

The ACA ratio is expressed here as a single number rather than as a ratio for simplicity, since the denominator is always 1. Thus, 6Δ/D is equivalent to 6Δ:1D.

BINOCULAR VISION SYNDROMES

Duane described four types of binocular vision syndromes: convergence insufficiency, convergence excess, divergence insufficiency, and divergence excess.[2,6] These syndromes have been defined in somewhat different ways by different investigators. A clinically useful description of the syndromes based on the phoria findings characteristic of each is given in Table 2.1. The phoria lines typical of each are shown in Figure 2.4. Convergence insufficiency and divergence insufficiency are characterized by low stimulus ACA ratios; convergence excess and divergence excess are characterized by high ratios. The syndromes will be discussed in more detail later.

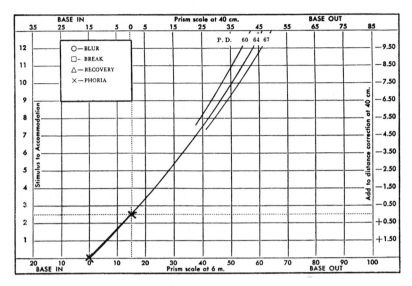

Figure 2.3 The phoria line falls on the demand line for an individual with orthophoria at 6 m and orthophoria at 40 cm (both phorias through the subjective refraction). The stimulus ACA ratio is thus 6.

Table 2.1
Findings characteristic of Duane's binocular vision syndromes.

	Distance Phoria	*Near Phoria*
Convergence insufficiency	Approximate orthophoria	High exophoria
Convergence excess	Approximate orthophoria	Esophoria
Divergence insufficiency	Esophoria	Low exophoria or approximate orthophoria
Divergence excess	High exophoria	Low exophoria or approximate orthophoria

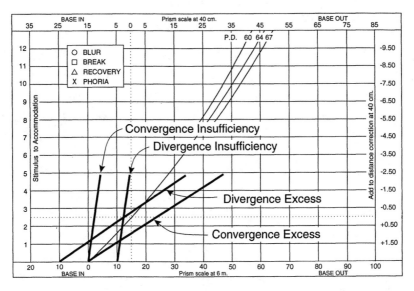

Figure 2.4 Examples of phoria lines representing Duane's four binocular vision syndromes. Although the examples represent four individuals, they are plotted together for illustrative purposes.

REFERENCES

1. Cline D, Hofstetter HW, Griffin JR. *Dictionary of Visual Science.* 4th ed. Radnor, PA: Chilton; 1989:525.
2. Alpern M. Types of movement. In: Davson H, ed. *Muscular Mechanisms.* 2nd ed. Vol 3 of *The Eye.* New York, NY: Academic Press; 1969:65–174.
3. Morgan MW. The Maddox analysis of vergence. In: Schor CM, Ciuffreda KJ, eds. *Vergence Eye Movements: Basic and Clinical Aspects.* Boston, MA: Butterworth-Heinemann; 1983:15–21.
4. Moses RA. Accommodation. In: Moses RA, Hart WM Jr, eds. *Adler's Physiology of the Eye.* 8th ed. St Louis, MO: Mosby; 1987:291–310.
5. Thompson HS. The pupil. In: Moses RA, Hart WM Jr, eds. *Adler's Physiology of the Eye.* 8th ed. St Louis, MO: Mosby; 1987:311–338.
6. Wick BC. Horizontal deviations. In: Amos JF, ed. *Diagnosis and Management in Vision Care.* Boston, MA: Butterworth-Heinemann; 1987:461–510.

SUGGESTED READING

Hofstetter HW. The graphical analysis of clinical optometric findings. In: *Transactions of the International Ophthalmic Optical Congress 1961.* London, UK: Lockwood, 1962:456–460.
Pitts DG, Hofstetter HW. Demand-line graphing of the zone of clear single binocular vision. *Am Optom Assoc J.* 1959:31:51–55.

PRACTICE PROBLEMS

1. For the patients in the following table, plot the phorias, draw the phoria lines, and determine the calculated and gradient ACA ratios.

	Patient AD 60-mm PD	Patient EJ 64-mm PD	Patient TB 64-mm PD	Patient SP 67-mm PD	Patient GP 63-mm PD
Phoria at 6 m through subjective refraction	1 exophoria	1 esophoria	0	2 esophoria	0
Phoria at 40 cm through subjective refraction		4 exophoria	2 exophoria	4 esophoria	9 exophoria
Phoria at 40 cm through a +1.00 add over subjective refraction		7 exophoria			
Phoria at 33 cm through subjective refraction	2 exophoria		2 exophoria		

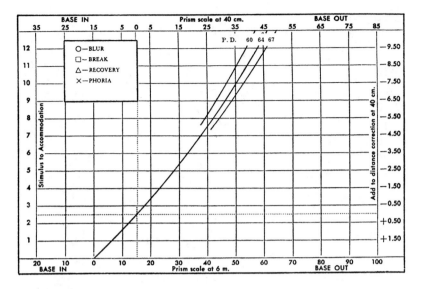

Patient AD

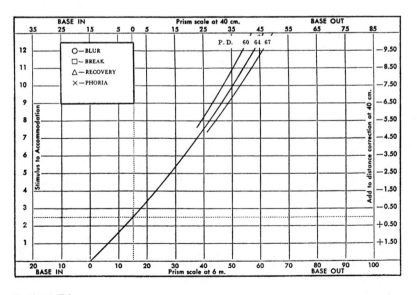

Patient EJ

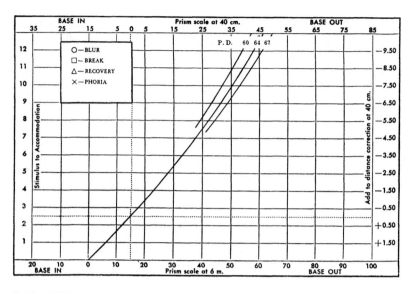

Patient TB

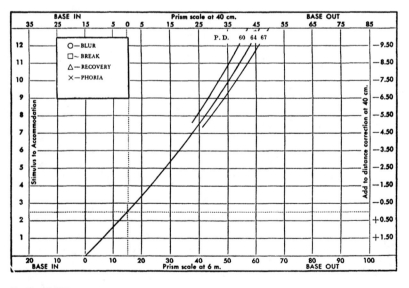

Patient SP

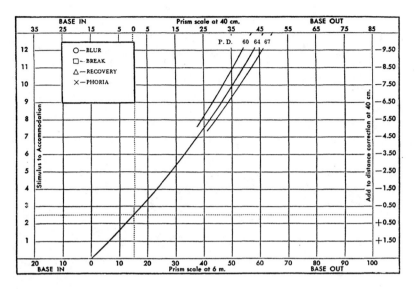

Patient GP

2. Using the data in Figures 2.1, 2.2, and 2.3, calculate stimulus ACA ratios as many ways as you can. Do your calculated values agree with your estimated values from the graphs?
3. Graph the phorias and draw the phoria lines for the findings given as examples in the text section on calculating stimulus ACA ratios (pp 12–13).

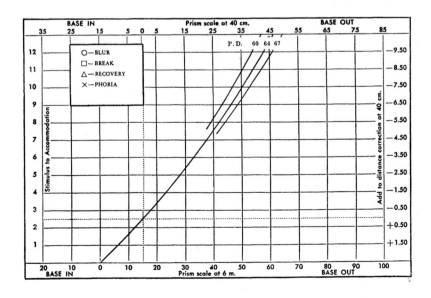

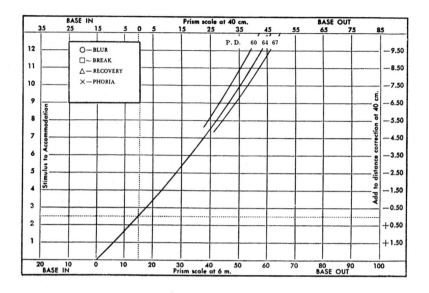

3

Plotting Blur, Break, Recovery, and Amplitude Findings and Completing Graphs

This chapter will describe how the rest of the findings used in graphical analysis are plotted on the graph and how erroneous findings are detected. It also will examine some characteristics of the completed graph.

PLOTTING BASE-IN AND BASE-OUT FINDINGS

The base-in and base-out to blur, break, and recovery findings are plotted in the same manner as for phorias but with different symbols. Follow the steps listed below to plot these findings:

1. Find the point on the demand line for the given testing distance.
2. Go straight up one space for each diopter of minus added to the distance subjective refraction or go straight down one space for each diopter of plus over the subjective.
3. Move to the right one space for each 10Δ of base-out or to the left one space for each 10Δ of base-in.
4. Mark blurs with circles, breaks with squares, and recoveries with triangles.

PLOTTING PLUS- AND MINUS-TO-BLUR FINDINGS

After adding plus spheres binocularly to the first sustained blur and then minus spheres binocularly to the first sustained blur, plot the findings as follows:

1. Find the point on the demand line corresponding to the testing distance.
2. If the test was performed through prisms, move to the right or left appropriately.

3. Move straight up one space for each diopter of minus added to the distance subjective correction or straight down one space for each diopter of plus added to the distance subjective correction. (If the test was started with lenses added to the subjective, include the difference in power from the subjective when moving up or down.)
4. Use a circle to mark the point at which a blur occurs. If a break occurs without a blur, use a square to mark the point.
5. Connect the base-in to blur and the base-in to break without blur findings with the minus-to-blur findings. Similarly connect the base-out to blur and the base-out to break without blur findings with the plus-to-blur findings.
6. If breaks beyond blurs are also plotted, interconnect all the breaks in the base-in direction with line segments to show the divergence limits and all the breaks in the base-out direction to show the convergence limits. Similarly interconnect the base-in and base-out recovery points to enclose the fusion recovery range at the various accommodative stimulus levels.

PLOTTING AMPLITUDE OF ACCOMMODATION

Amplitude of accommodation usually is measured by means of the push-up test, in which a target is brought closer and closer to the patient until the best visual acuity letters appear blurred to the patient. The stopping point is the first blur that cannot be cleared. The test generally is done with the patient wearing the exact correction for his or her ametropia or, for the presbyope, with some added plus. The distance (near-point of accommodation) is converted into diopters of stimulus to accommodation, with any amount of plus over the subjective refraction worn during the test subtracted or any minus added. For example, if a near-point of accommodation of 33 cm with unaided vision is obtained and the patient is subsequently found to be a 1.00D hyperope, the amplitude of accommodation is $1/0.33\text{m} + 1.00D = 4.00D$. Similarly, if a near-point of accommodation of 20 cm is measured for a myope wearing the habitual prescription of $-1.50D$ sph OU and the subjective refraction is $-2.25D$ sph OU, the amplitude of accommodation is $1/0.2 \text{ m} - 0.75D = 4.25D$.

A formula that incorporates the difference in the power of the lenses through which the patient was tested (test lenses) and the patient's distance subjective refraction (refractive error) and that uses centimeters as the unit for near-point of accommodation (NPA) is as follows:

Amplitude of accommodation (in D) =

$$\frac{100}{NPA \text{ (in cm)}} - (\text{test lenses} - \text{refractive error})$$

Once the amplitude of accommodation has been calculated, a horizontal line is drawn across the graph, starting at the stimulus to accommodation level equal to the amplitude of accommodation. This line demarcates the top of the zone of clear single binocular vision (ZCSBV) on the graph.

CONVERGENCE AMPLITUDE

The convergence amplitude is determined with the near-point of convergence (NPC) test and the formula for convergence stimulus. To determine the NPC, a small object is brought toward the patient until the patient reports diplopia or until one eye swings out or fails to converge further as the object is brought nearer. The distance of this point from the spectacle plane is measured; this distance can then be added to 2.7 cm to obtain the value d in the following formula:

$$\text{Convergence stimulus (in } \Delta) = \frac{10 \times PD \text{ (in mm)}}{d \text{ (in cm)}}$$

For example, an individual with a 58-mm PD and a 6-cm NPC will have a convergence amplitude of

$$\frac{10 \times 58 \text{ mm}}{6 \text{ cm} + 2.7 \text{ cm}} = \frac{580}{8.7} = 66.7\Delta$$

A person with a 64-mm PD and a 7-cm NPC will have a convergence amplitude of

$$\frac{10 \times 64 \text{ mm}}{7 \text{ cm} + 2.7 \text{ cm}} = \frac{640}{9.7} = 66.0\Delta$$

To mark convergence amplitude on the graph, find the value of the convergence amplitude on the base-out side of the 6-m prism scale and draw a vertical line through that point. Alternatively, a vertical line can be drawn through the point on the demand line corresponding to the NPC. In most instances, however, as in the two examples, the convergence amplitude will exceed the maximum demand line value provided for on the standard graph.

ZONE OF CLEAR SINGLE BINOCULAR VISION

The graph is now ready for completion. The most convergent base-out to blur value or base-out to break without blur value should be connected with the point of intersection of the convergence and accommodative amplitude lines. In the absence of either of the two amplitude lines, the trend of the base-out to blur limits should be continued as a dashed line obliquely up and to the right until it reaches the other amplitude line. In principle, the positive fusional convergence border and the convergence and accommodative amplitude lines have a common intersection. Similarly, the base-out to break beyond the blur values can be extended to the point of intersection of the convergence and accommodative amplitude lines.

The trends of the phorias and the base-in blurs, breaks, and recoveries can all be extended obliquely upward as dashed lines to the accommodative amplitude line at slopes approximating their respective line-segment slopes at the lower accommodative levels.

The ZCSBV is the area within the blur lines, the amplitude lines, and the base line on the bottom of the graph through 0 stimulus to accommodation. Figures 3.1 and 3.2 provide examples of completed graphs.

The ZCSBV represents the area in which the patient can see clearly and singly. It predicts how the patient will respond to different viewing distances, lenses, and prisms. To better understand the nature of the ZCSBV, we can relate five of its geometric properties to clinical correlates[1-3]:

1. The lateral position of the graph corresponds to the distance phoria.
2. The height of the zone corresponds to the amplitude of accommodation.
3. The correlate of the slope of the zone is the reciprocal of the stimulus ACA ratio.
4. The positive width corresponds to positive fusional convergence, the lateral distance from the phoria line to the base-out boundary.
5. The negative width represents negative fusional convergence, the lateral distance from the phoria line to the base-in boundary.

The five geometric properties of the ZCSBV are illustrated in Figure 3.3.

Detection of Erroneous Findings

If we do not consider for the moment variability in lateral position, slope, height, and widths of the ZCSBV, we can describe its general form (which is also shown in Figure 3.4):

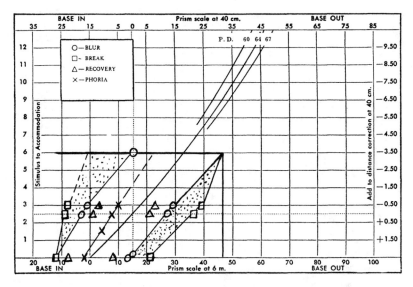

Figure 3.1 A completed graph, with the dotted areas indicating single but blurred vision. The numerical findings are given in the following table. All the findings are taken through the subjective refraction unless otherwise noted.

	Phoria	Base-in	Base-out	Plus-to-Blur	Minus-to-Blur
6 m	2 exophoria	X/12/8	13/21/8		
40 cm	7 exophoria	19/24/14	12/19/7	+2.25	−3.50
33 cm	8 exophoria	19/26/13	11/21/6		
40 cm through +1.00 over subjective	11 exophoria				

Near-point of accommodation, 17 cm; NPC, 11 cm; PD, 65 mm.

1. The phoria line is expected to approximate a straight line.
2. The line formed by the base-in to blur (or base-in to break if no blur is obtained) and minus-to-blur findings is expected to be parallel to the phoria line. It should be approximately straight, but may have a short vertical portion at the bottom and a slight curve at the top.
3. The line connecting the base-out to blur (or base-out to break if no blur is obtained) and the plus-to-blur findings also should be

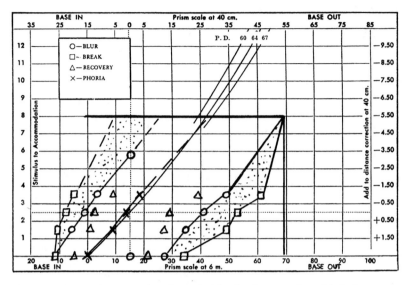

Figure 3.2 Another completed graph. The findings in the table below are taken through the subjective refraction unless otherwise noted.

	Phoria	Base-in	Base-out	Plus-to-Blur	Minus-to-Blur
6 m	Orthophoria	X/12/4	27/34/21		
40 cm	1 exophoria	16/23/13	26/38/14	+2.50	−3.25
40 cm + 1.00	6 exophoria	21/26/14	20/34/12		
40 cm − 1.00	3 esophoria	12/20/6	34/46/24		

Near-point of accommodation, 12.5 cm; NPC, 6.5 cm; PD, 63 mm.

    approximately straight and parallel to the phoria line. It may have a slight curve at the bottom and a short vertical segment at the top.

4. The ZCSBV should approximate a parallelogram.
5. Because of accommodative convergence, phoria and blur lines should tilt toward the right.

An individual finding can be considered probably erroneous if it deviates significantly from the pattern that otherwise conforms to the expected configuration. Such a finding can be the result of any of several factors. Errors are easy to identify if the findings are taken with a

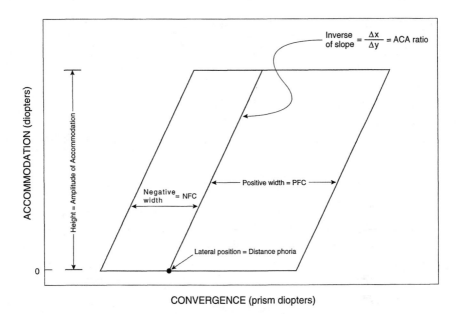

Figure 3.3 The five geometrical properties of the ZCSBV and their clinical correlates.

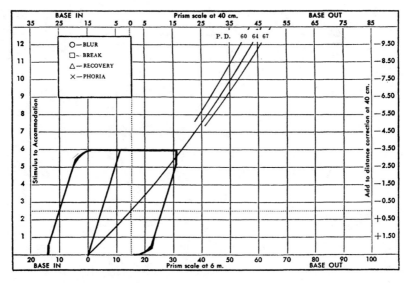

Figure 3.4 Typical form of boundaries of the ZCSBV without reference to lateral position, slope, height, or width.

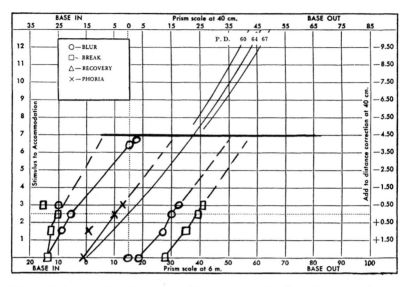

Figure 3.5 A graph with two possible erroneous findings. For easy viewing, only the blur, break, and phoria lines are plotted. The amplitude of accommodation is 7.00D; the rest of the findings are presented in the following table.

	Phoria	Base-in	Base-out	Plus-to-Blur	Minus-to-Blur
6 m	1 exophoria	X/14/8	19/28/12		
40 cm	5 exophoria	20/25/16	16/24/12	+2.50	−4.00
33 cm	5 exophoria	28/34/16	14/22/10		−3.75
40 cm + 1.00	14 exophoria	24/28/18	12/20/8		

The base-in to blur at 33 cm and the phoria at 40 cm with the +1.00 may be in error.

number of lens and test distance combinations. Figure 3.5 provides an example of the detection of erroneous test results.

PROXIMAL CONVERGENCE

One deviation from the expected graph form may occur with an individual who exhibits a large amount of proximal convergence.[4] In this case the ZCSBV will appear to fan out. That is, the base- in and minus-to-blur line and the base-out and plus-to-blur line will appear farther apart as the stimulus to accommodation level increases. Proximal convergence and the cause of this apparent aberration in the ZCSBV will be discussed in more detail in the next chapter.

REFERENCES

1. Fry GA. Fundamental variables in the relationship between accommodation and convergence. *Optom Weekly.* 1943;34:153– 155, 183–185.
2. Hofstetter HW. The zone of clear single binocular vision. *Am J Optom Arch Am Acad Optom.* 1945;22:301–333, 361–384.
3. Hofstetter HW. Graphical analysis. In: Schor CM, Ciuffreda KJ, eds. *Vergence Eye Movements: Basic and Clinical Aspects.* Boston, MA: Butterworth-Heinemann; 1983:439–464.
4. Hofstetter HW. The relationship of proximal convergence to fusional and accommodative convergence. *Am J Optom Arch Am Acad Optom.* 1951;28: 300–308.

SUGGESTED READING

Pitts DG, Hofstetter HW. Demand-line graphing of the zone of clear single binocular vision. *Am Optom Assoc J.* 1959;31:51– 55.

PRACTICE PROBLEMS

Graph the following information. All findings are taken with the subjective refraction in place unless otherwise indicated. For each patient, draw in the boundaries of the ZCSBV, determine whether there are any erroneous findings, and calculate the stimulus ACA ratio.

	Patient BP 62-mm PD	Patient AT 66-mm PD	Patient GP 64-mm PD	Patient DK 64-mm PD	Patient HF 60-mm PD
Near-point of accommodation	12.5 cm	20 cm	17 cm	10 cm	11 cm
NPC	5 cm	18 cm	11 cm	9 cm	9 cm
6 m phoria	2 esophoria	3 exophoria			orthophoria
6 m base-in	X/15/8	X/16/8			X/8/4
6 m base-out	28/38/20	12/16/12			10/18/8
4 m phoria			1 exophoria	4 exophoria	
4 m base-in			X/10/6	X/12/4	
4 m base-out			20/28/16	12/20/6	
40 cm phoria	5 esophoria	11 exophoria	5 exophoria	8 exophoria	10 exophoria
40 cm base-in	14/22/10	26/30/20	16/22/8	18/24/6	20/23/18
40 cm base-out	32/42/24	6/14/2	16/24/12	12/24/8	6/14/2
40 cm plus-to-blur	+2.50	+2.00	+2.50	+2.00	+1.50
40 cm minus-to-blur	−1.00	−2.50	−3.50	−5.25	−6.50
40 cm + 1.00 add phoria	3 exophoria		9 exophoria	12 exophoria	11 exophoria
40 cm + 1.00 add base-in	18/26/12		22/24/8	24/28/12	
40 cm + 1.00 add base-out	26/34/18		10/18/2	18/22/2	
33 cm phoria		13 exophoria		9 exophoria	
33 cm base-in		28/36/20			
33 cm base-out		7/12/4			
33 cm plus-to-blur		+3.00			
33 cm minus-to-blur		−2.00			

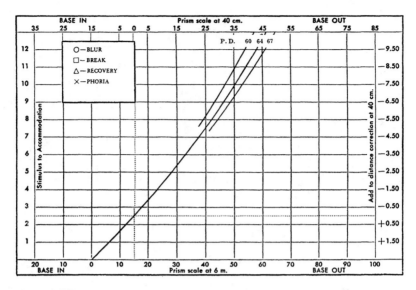

Patient BP

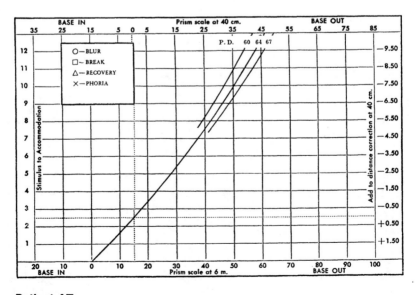

Patient AT

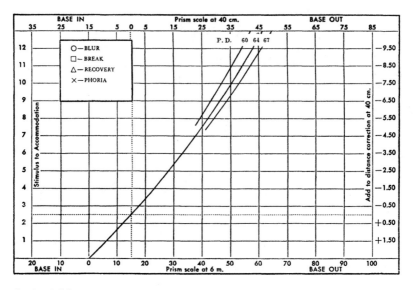

Patient GP

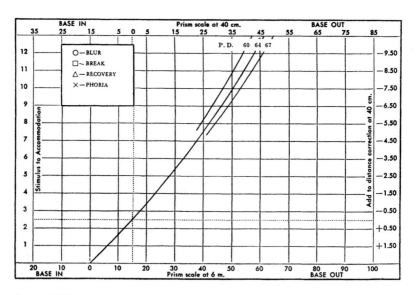

Patient DK

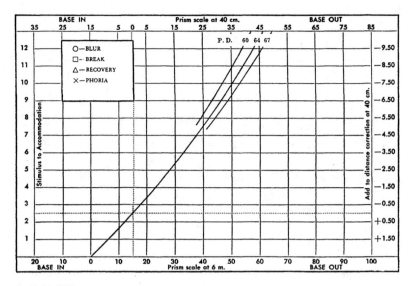

Patient HF

4

Effects of Lag of Accommodation and Proximal Convergence on the Zone of Clear Single Binocular Vision

In Chapter 3 we saw that the expected shape of the zone of clear single binocular vision (ZCSBV) is a parallelogram. With the inclusion of the phoria line it becomes a double parallelogram. Two common causes of departure from this expected form are lag of accommodation and proximal convergence.

LAG OF ACCOMMODATION

Clinically we try to assure that the accommodative response will be approximately equal to the accommodative stimulus by instructing the patient to keep the test letters clear. Because of the depth of focus, the accommodative response does not have to exactly equal the stimulus to accommodation for clear vision. For example, if the depth of focus is 1.00D and the patient is wearing the correction for ametropia, the accommodative response can vary from approximately 2.00D to approximately 3.00D while target clarity is retained at 40 cm. For most individuals the accommodative response tends to be less than the stimulus to accommodation; this is referred to as the "lag of accommodation." Sheard[1] was the first to describe the lag.

The ACA ratio that would most closely describe the physiologic interaction of accommodative convergence and accommodation would be the ratio of the amount of accommodative convergence to the corresponding change in accommodative response. This is called the "response ACA ratio" and it can be determined if accommodative response is measured by an optometer or a retinoscopic arrangement. Clinically, we know the accommodative stimulus from the test distance and the test lenses used, but we usually do not measure the accommodative response. As a result, the ACA ratio derived clinically usually is the ratio of the amount of accommodative convergence to the corresponding change in stimulus to accommodation ("stimulus ACA ratio").

The stimulus ACA ratio will not equal the response ACA ratio if the lag of accommodation changes. The lag of accommodation can be minimized by requiring the patient to view letters close to his or her best visual acuity and to keep the letters clear. In fact, the single most common source of error in clinically measured phorias and ACA ratios is the failure to include this requirement.

A lag of accommodation that is variable or that increases with stimulus to accommodation can be detected by noting a phoria line that is tipped less toward the abscissa (thus indicating a lower ACA ratio) than are the base-in and base-out limit lines. If there is a large lag of accommodation at the higher stimulus to accommodation, calculation of the stimulus ACA ratio will yield a lower value than is actually the case. An example is provided in Figure 4.1. Cases with findings similar to those in Figure 4.1 have been called "false convergence insufficiency" or "pseudoconvergence insufficiency."[2,3] Pseudoconvergence insufficiency is more of an accommodative problem than a convergence problem, so common treatments are plus adds or vision training to improve accommodative function.[2-5]

PROXIMAL CONVERGENCE

Proximal convergence is convergence caused by awareness of nearness of a target.[6] Individuals who exhibit a great deal of proximal convergence have a characteristic alteration in the ZCSBV. The zone appears to fan out; that is, it is wider at the higher stimulus to accommodation. This is due to the fact that the base-out findings are affected the most by proximal convergence and the base-in findings are affected the least, with the phorias falling somewhere in between.[7] One way to demonstrate this is to obtain one set of findings at distance with different minus adds over the subjective refraction and another set of findings at near-point with plus adds over the subjective refraction. The two sets of data will thus have used the same levels of stimulus of accommodation but different test distances.

If the subject in this experiment happens to show proximal convergence, results like those shown in Figures 4.2 and 4.3 will be obtained. In Figure 4.2 the lines connecting points for 6-m test distance findings are separate from the lines connecting 33-cm findings. In Figure 4.3

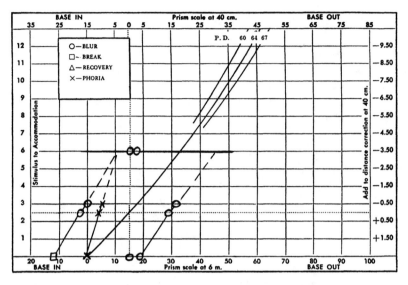

Figure 4.1 Effects of lag of accommodation. The findings in the following table are plotted in the graph. The examiner did not require the patient to keep letters clear while performing the phorias. As a result, the phoria line is not parallel to the base-in and base-out limit lines. The ACA ratio is thus evidently higher than the phoria line indicates. The syndrome typified by this set of findings has been called "false" or "pseudoconvergence insufficiency." Besides procedural inadequacy, it also may indicate an accommodative dysfunction.

	Phoria	Base-in	Base-out	Plus-to-Blur	Minus-to-Blur
6 m	Orthophoria	X/12/6	18/24/16		
40 cm	11 exophoria	18/28/12	14/20/16	+2.50	−3.50
33 cm	13 exophoria	18/26/16	15/22/12		−3.00

lines connect the points that more closely represent a typical clinical routine. In the same figure the base-in and base-out boundaries of the ZCSBV fan out.

In Figure 4.2 the two base-out lines are separated more than the two phoria lines, which in turn are separated more than the two base-in findings. This agrees with the hierarchy mentioned earlier for the findings most affected by proximal convergence. Hofstetter[7] found that for a group of 21 young adult subjects in an experiment similar to the one shown in Figures 4.2 and 4.3, the average amounts of displace-

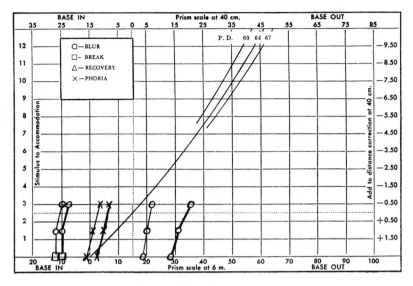

Figure 4.2 To demonstrate proximal convergence, base-in and base-out limits and phorias were taken at 6 m (thin lines) and 33 cm (heavy lines) with various adds over the subjective refraction. The data are given in the following table.

	Phoria	Base-in Limit	Base-out Limit
6 m	1 exophoria	12	18
6 m − 1.50	2 esophoria	11	20
6 m − 3.00	4 esophoria	9	22
33 cm	10 exophoria	27	18
33 cm + 1.50	12 exophoria	29	14
33 cm + 3.00	14 exophoria	30	12

ment of the base-in, phoria, and base-out lines were 1.5Δ, 2.6Δ, and 7.6Δ, respectively.

One possible explanation for differing amounts of proximal convergence on the base-out, phoria, and base-in lines is that perception of distance changes as prism power is added under binocular conditions. As base-out prism power is increased, the target seems to get closer. As base-in prism power is increased, the target seems to get farther away. A related observation is that proximal convergence is greater under conditions of binocular fusion than under unfused conditions.[8]

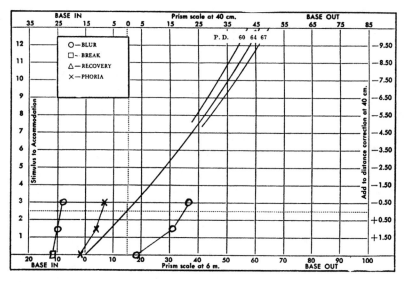

Figure 4.3 Effects of proximal convergence. This figure plots the findings from the previous figure taken at 6 m through the subjective and at 33 cm through the subjective and with a +1.50D add over the subjective. The findings are somewhat representative of a typical set of clinical findings. The zone fans out, a characteristic configuration for an individual who exhibits a typical amount of proximal convergence.

REFERENCES

1. Sheard C. Dynamic skiametry and methods of testing the accommodation and convergence of the eyes. In: *The Sheard Volume—Selected Writings in Visual and Ophthalmic Optics.* Philadelphia, PA: Chilton; 1957:125–230 (originally published as a monograph in 1920).
2. Grosvenor TP. *Primary Care Optometry.* 2nd ed. Boston, MA: Butterworth-Heinemann; 1989:345–346.
3. Richman JE, Cron MT. *Guide to Vision Therapy.* South Bend, IN: Bernell Corp; 1987:17–18.
4. Heath GG. The use of graphic analysis in visual training. *Am J Optom Arch Am Acad Optom.* 1959;36:337–350.
5. Mazow ML, France TD, Finkelman S, et al. Acute accommodative and convergence insufficiency. *Trans Am Ophthalmol Soc.* 1989;87:158–173.
6. Hofstetter HW. The proximal factor in accommodation and convergence. *Am J Optom Arch Am Acad Optom.* 1942;19:67–76.
7. Hofstetter HW. The relationship of proximal convergence to fusional and accommodative convergence. *Am J Optom Arch Am Acad Optom.* 1951;28:300–308.
8. Wick B. Clinical factors in proximal vergence. *Am J Optom Physiol Opt.* 1985;62:1–18.

SUGGESTED READING

Alpern M. Types of movement. In: Davson H, ed. *Muscular Mechanisms*. 2nd ed. Vol 3 of *The Eye*. New York, NY: Academic; 1969:65–174 (see especially pp 141–143).

Ciuffreda KJ, Kenyon RV. Accommodative vergence and accommodation in normals, amblyopes, and strabismics. In: Schor CM, Ciuffreda KJ, eds. *Vergence Eye Movements: Basic and Clinical Aspects*. Boston, MA: Butterworth-Heinemann; 1983:101–173 (see especially pp 101–103).

Hokoda SC, Ciuffreda KJ. Theoretical and clinical importance of proximal vergence and accommodation. In: Schor CM, Ciuffreda KJ, eds. *Vergence Eye Movements: Basic and Clinical Aspects*. Boston, MA: Butterworth-Heinemann; 1983: 75–97 (see especially pp 90–92).

PRACTICE PROBLEMS

1. Why would the gradient ACA ratio not be affected by proximal convergence?
2. Which would you expect to be higher in a person exhibiting considerable proximal convergence: the gradient ACA ratio or the calculated ACA ratio? Explain.
3. Would the stimulus ACA ratio equal the response ACA ratio if the lag of accommodation were constant during all phoria measurements? Explain.

5

Definitions of Terms

TYPES OF VERGENCE

To aid in theoretical and clinical thinking, it is useful to classify vergences into types. The early classification scheme of Maddox[1-3] provides a helpful framework. In this scheme vergence eye movements are described as tonic, accommodative, proximal, and fusional. "Tonic convergence" represents the result of tonus in the extraocular muscles; that is, it is the physiologic position of rest of the eyes. The clinical correlate of the combination of tonic convergence and the anatomic position of rest of the eyes is the distance phoria through the subjective refraction. Thus, the distance phoria is said to represent tonic convergence. "Accommodative convergence" is convergence that occurs as part of the synkinesis of convergence and accommodation. The ACA ratio is the accommodative convergence in prism diopters per diopter of accommodation. "Proximal, or psychic, convergence" is convergence caused by the awareness of nearness of a given object of fixation. "Fusional convergence" serves to maintain fusion of the two retinal images. "Disparity vergence" often is used as a synonym for fusional convergence because the effective stimulus for these movements is retinal disparity.[4-6]

Maddox's writings were based on clinical experience rather than controlled experimentation.[3] Maddox's concepts are an oversimplification of the physiology of vergence eye movements, but the Maddox classification is a useful construct that aids in understanding clinical analysis of convergence.

The above terms describing the Maddox classification of vergence have been defined earlier; they appear here for the sake of review and to prevent confusion with the terms soon to be discussed. The nomenclature is based on theoretical stimulus or response correlates of the particular movements. The terms to be covered next are clinical constructs used to describe the results of testing accommodation and convergence. They can be easily visualized by means of graphical analysis.[7,8]

TERMS USED IN CLINICAL TESTING

The "positive relative convergence" (PRC) at a given level of accommodation is the horizontal distance on the graph from the demand line to the right-hand limit of the zone of clear single binocular vision (ZCSBV). The "negative relative convergence" (NRC) is the horizontal distance from the demand line to the left-hand limit of the ZCSBV. For testing done with the subjective refraction lenses in place, the NRC and PRC are the base-in and base-out limits, respectively, as read from the Risley prisms. (The base-in and base-out limits are the blur findings with increasing prism or the break findings if no blur occurs.) The "positive fusional convergence" (PFC) for a given stimulus to accommodation level is the horizontal distance on the graph from the phoria line to the right-hand boundary of the ZCSBV. The "negative fusional convergence" (NFC) is the horizontal distance from the phoria line to the left-hand boundary of the ZCSBV.

The phoria test is a measure of the amount of fusional convergence required for single binocular vision at the testing distance. Thus, for a given test distance, the "demand on fusional convergence" is equal to the horizontal distance on the graph from the phoria line to the demand line. When the phoria is taken through the patient's ametropic correction, the demand is equal to the phoria.

The "reserve" is the horizontal distance from the demand line to the right-hand limit of the ZCSBV in exophoria and to the left-hand limit in esophoria. It represents the amount of fusional convergence that can still be exerted after the demand has been met. In exophoria the reserve also is called the "positive fusional reserve convergence" (PFRC), and it is equal to the PRC. In esophoria the reserve also is called the "negative fusional reserve convergence" (NFRC), and it is equal to the difference between the NFC and the demand. The NFRC is also equivalent to the NRC.

Examples of the graphical dimensions associated with these terms are presented in Figures 5.1 and 5.2. Figure 5.1 shows the graph for a patient with an exophoria of 4Δ at 40 cm. The vergence posture of the eyes during the measurement of the near phoria is dependent on tonic, proximal, and accommodative convergence. The PFC and NFC represent the fusional convergence that can be exerted in the convergent (base-out) and divergent (base-in) directions, respectively, from that point. The PRC and NRC are measurements of the patient's convergence and divergence capabilities with respect to the target; on the graph they are measured from a point on the demand line corresponding to the testing distance. Figure 5.2 illustrates an example showing near-point esophoria. The following formulas give the relationship of fusional convergence and relative convergence values:

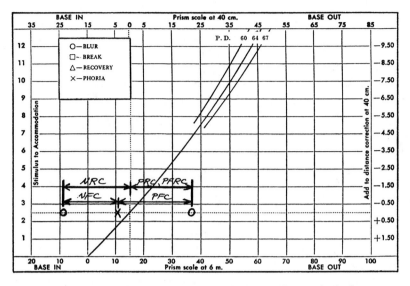

Figure 5.1 At 40 cm for a given individual, an exophoria of 4Δ along with a base-in blur of 24 and a base-out blur of 22 are measured. Thus, the NRC is 24, the NFC is 20, the PFC is 26, the PRC is 22, and the PFRC is 22.

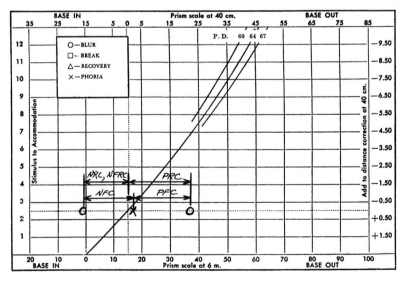

Figure 5.2 At 40 cm for another individual, an esophoria of 2Δ is measured. The base-in and base-out blur findings are 16 and 22, respectively. Therefore, the NRC is 16, the NFC is 18, the NFRC is 16, the PRC is 22, and the PFC is 20.

PFC = PRC − phoria

NFC = NRC + phoria

Exophoria is a minus value in the formulas and esophoria is a plus since they represent divergent and convergent positions, respectively, in relation to the target.

Figures 5.3 and 5.4 give illustrative examples of locations of the lines of sight during tests. Figure 5.3 shows the lines of sight for distance testing for a patient with esophoria. Figure 5.4 shows an example of exophoria at near and the base-in and base-out limits.

The "positive relative accommodation" (PRA) is the vertical distance upward on the graph from the demand line to the boundary of the ZCSBV. The "negative relative accommodation" (NRA) is the vertical distance downward on the graph from the demand line to the border of the

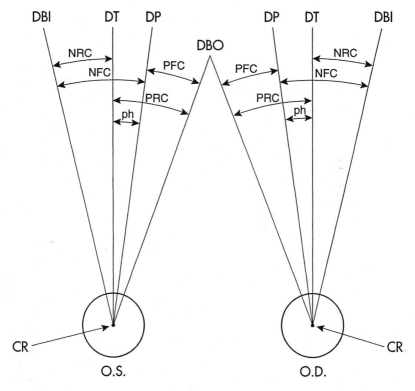

Figure 5.3 Positions of the lines of sight of the eyes during various tests for a patient with esophoria at distance. CR, center of rotation; DBI, position at distance base-in break; DT, position if target is fused at infinity (parallelism of the lines of sight); DP, distance phoria position; DBO, position at distance base-out blur; ph, dissociated phoria.

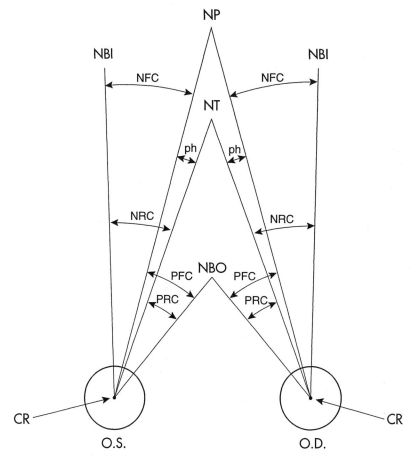

Figure 5.4 Positions of the lines of sight of the eyes during various tests for a patient with exophoria at near. CR, center of rotation; NBI, position at near base-in blur; NP, near phoria position; NT, position of near-point test target; NBO, position at near base-out blur; ph, dissociated phoria.

zone. The NRA and the PRA represent the binocular plus-lens-to-blur test and the binocular minus-lens-to-blur test, respectively, when these tests are both started with the subjective refraction in place (Figure 5.5).

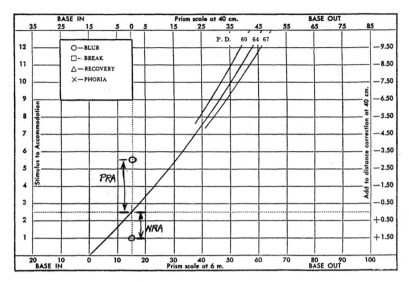

Figure 5.5 The NRA and PRA at 40 cm for a patient with a plus-to-blur of +1.50D and a minus-to-blur of −3.00D.

REFERENCES

1. Maddox EE. *The Clinical Use of Prisms; and the Decentration of Lenses.* 2nd ed. Bristol, England: John Wright & Co; 1893:83–106.
2. Schor C. Introduction to the symposium on basic and clinical aspects of vergence eye movements. *Am J Optom Physiol Opt.* 1980;57:535–536.
3. Morgan MW. The Maddox analysis of vergence. In: Schor CM, Ciuffreda KJ, eds. *Vergence Eye Movements: Basic and Clinical Aspects.* Boston, MA: Butterworth-Heinemann; 1983:15–21.
4. Stark L, Kenyon RV, Krishnan VV, Ciuffreda KJ. Disparity vergence: a proposed name for a dominant component of binocular vergence eye movements. *Am J Optom Physiol Opt.* 1980;57:606–669.
5. Fry GA. Disparity vergence. *Am J Optom Physiol Opt.* 1981;58:685. Letter to the Editor.
6. Stark L. Reply. *Am J Optom Physiol Opt.* 1981; 58:686. Letter to the Editor.
7. Hofstetter HW. The graphical analysis of clinical optometric findings. In: *Transactions of the International Ophthalmic Optical Congress 1961.* London, UK: Lockwood; 1962:456–460.
8. Hofstetter HW. Graphical analysis. In: Schor CM, Ciuffreda KJ, eds. *Vergence Eye Movements: Basic and Clinical Aspects.* Boston, MA: Butterworth-Heinemann; 1983:439–464.

SUGGESTED READING

Michaels DD. *Visual Optics and Refraction—A Clinical Approach.* 3rd ed. St Louis, MO: Mosby; 1985:361–365.

PRACTICE PROBLEM

For the patients in the practice problems section of Chapter 3, determine the NRC, PRC, NFC, PFC, and NFRC or PFRC at distance and at 40 cm through the subjective refraction. For the same patients, determine the NRA and PRA values at 40 cm.

6

Sheard's Criterion

Of the various analytical criteria for evaluating lateral imbalances, the most widely used is Sheard's criterion.[1,2] The work of Hofstetter[3] suggested that application of Sheard's criterion correlates well with asthenopic symptoms and with relief of symptoms by convergence training. This was confirmed by Sheedy and Saladin,[4,5] who found that of several convergence and fixation disparity criteria, Sheard's criterion was the most effective in predicting asthenopic symptoms, and by Dalziel,[6] who reported that vision training that brought convergence findings to the point at which Sheard's criterion was met was effective in alleviating symptoms.

Sheard's postulate was that the fusional reserve should be at least twice the demand. Thus, the positive fusional reserve convergence should be at least twice the amount of an exophoria and the negative fusional reserve convergence should be at least twice the amount of an esophoria. A mathematical expression to describe this is $R \geq 2D$, where R represents the reserve and D represents the demand. To determine how much prism correction is necessary to allow Sheard's criterion to just be met at a given distance, we can use any of three methods: (1) trial and error substitution of values into the formula $R = 2D$, (2) inspection of the graph, or (3) the formula $P = 2/3D - 1/3R$, where P represents the required prism. (In this formula D is always positive regardless of whether an exophoria or an esophoria is present, and R is always positive whether positive relative convergence is used, as in exophoria, or negative relative convergence is used, as in esophoria.) When P equals 0 or a negative number, Sheard's criterion is met without any prism correction. A positive number indicates that prism is necessary for the criterion to be met: base-in prism in exophoria or base-out prism in esophoria.

In addition to using prism correction, Sheard's criterion also can be met by a change in the spherical lens power from the subjective or by vision training. The dioptric amount by which lens power must be altered from the distance subjective is given by the formula $S = P/A$, where S represents the spherical lens change, P represents the prism correction in the earlier formula, and A represents the ACA ratio. The purpose of this formula is to find the lens addition power that reduces the phoria enough to allow Sheard's criterion to be met. The gradient

ACA ratio is a measure of the amount of vergence change associated with 1D of accommodation change. This formula uses the gradient ACA ratio (A) to determine the spherical lens power change (S) that would change the phoria an amount equal to P. In this formula P is negative if base-in prism is necessary to meet Sheard's criterion; P is positive for base-out prism. Since a decrease in plus power or an increase in minus power increases accommodation and thus also increases accommodative convergence, this approach is used in exophoria. Conversely, an increase in plus power or a decrease in minus power is used in esophoria. Since Sheard's criterion can be met some distances and not at others, a bifocal may at times be useful in this regard.

If Sheard's criterion is not met in exophoria, orthoptic vision training may be used to extend the right-hand boundary of the zone. In esophoria the left-hand border of the zone of clear single binocular vision would need to be extended. One can calculate the amount to which the reserve would have to be increased simply by doubling the phoria (the demand).

EXAMPLES OF THE USE OF SHEARD'S CRITERION

The rationale for prescription decisions will be developed in more detail later. Here we will look at some examples that illustrate how Sheard's criterion is used.

In the first example, shown in Figure 6.1, exophoria is measured at both distance and near. Sheard's criterion is met at 6 m but not at 40 cm, since the base-out blur at 40 cm (12 exophoria) is not twice the phoria (10 exophoria). To determine the prism correction necessary to meet Sheard's criterion at 40 cm we use the following formula:

$$P = 2/3D - 1/3R$$
$$= 2/3(10) - 1/3(12)$$
$$= 2\ 2/3\Delta \text{ base-in}$$

Base-in prism is used since the phoria is in the exo direction. To determine the lens change at 40 cm to meet Sheard's criterion, we need to calculate the gradient ACA ratio and then use the appropriate formula for the spherical lens change.

Gradient ACA ratio $= 12 - 10 = 2\Delta/D$

The gradient ACA ratio is 2, so we set A = 2 in the formula. Base-in prism would be used to meet Sheard's criterion, so P is negative in the following formula:

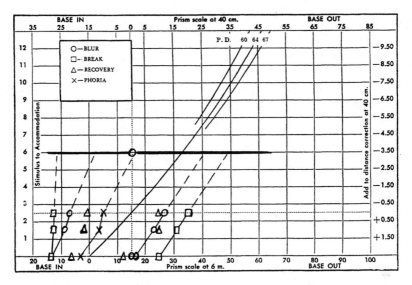

Figure 6.1 The test results in the following table are plotted in this graph.

	Phoria	Base-in	Base-out	Plus-to-Blur	Minus-to-Blur
6 m	3 exophoria	X/14/6	16/24/12		
40 cm	10 exophoria	22/28/16	12/20/10	+2.50	−3.50
40 cm + 1.00	12 exophoria	24/28/17	8/16/10		

Amplitude of accommodation = 6.00D.

$$S = P/A$$
$$= (-2.67\Delta)/(2\Delta/D)$$
$$= -1.34 \, D$$

The spherical lens change required at 40 cm to meet Sheard's criterion is −1.34D. The sign is minus because of the exo direction of the phoria, the minus reducing the exophoria by means of accommodative convergence. Another alternative is to increase the base-out blur to at least 20 by orthoptic vision training. In this type of situation, if there are complaints of asthenopia, the usual treatment is to prescribe base-out vision training or base-in prism for use at near. Although mathematically permissible, the prescription of excess minus sphere for exophoria is in disfavor clinically; the equivalent undercorrection of hyperopia is frequently acceptable, however, especially in the presence of ample accommodative ability.

Figure 6.2 illustrates a case of esophoria at distance and near. Sheard's criterion is met at 6 m but not at 40 cm or 33 cm. That is, at 40 cm and at 33 cm the reserve (base-in blur) is not twice the demand (phoria). Sheard's criterion would be fulfilled at 40 cm with the following prism:

$$P = 2/3D - 1/3R$$
$$= 2/3(12) - 1/3(12)$$
$$= 4\Delta \text{ base-out}$$

Base-out prism is required because of the esophoria.

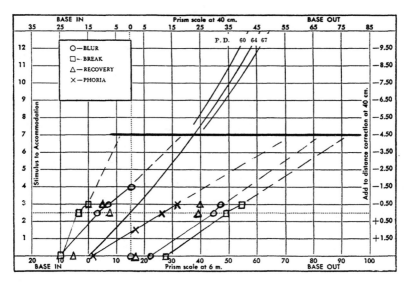

Figure 6.2 This figure illustrates the clinical findings given in the following table.

	Phoria	Base-in	Base-out	Plus-to-Blur	Minus-to-Blur
6 m	2 esophoria	X/10/6	22/28/16		
40 cm	12 esophoria	12/18/8	30/34/24	+2.50	−1.50
33 cm	14 esophoria	10/18/12	30/36/22		
40 cm + 1.00	2 esophoria				

Amplitude of accommodation = 7.00D.

Figure 6.2 indicates that the ACA ratio is quite high. The gradient ACA ratio is 10Δ/D P:

Gradient ACA ratio = $12 - 2 = 10\Delta$/D

Next we can substitute the gradient ACA ratio for A in the formula for spherical lens change. Base-out prism was required to meet Sheard's criterion so P is a positive number in the formula for spherical lens addition power.

S = P/A

   = $(+4\Delta)/(10\Delta$/D)

   = +0.40D

To reduce accommodative convergence and thus reduce the amount of esophoria, a plus lens change over the subjective refraction is indicated for near. Alternatively, vision training can be instituted to increase the base-in limit to at least 24 at 40 cm. The usual method of handling this type of case is to provide a plus add at near.

EFFECTIVENESS OF SHEARD'S CRITERION

Sheard's criterion should not be viewed as an exact, mathematically derived formula, but as a useful diagnostic aid or guideline. The studies cited in the first paragraph of this chapter and clinical experience show that Sheard's criterion is a useful clinical rule of thumb. Sheedy and Saladin[4,5] found Sheard's criterion to be the best predictor of ocular symptoms overall and especially in exo deviations, but other measures were more predictive in esophoria. Sheard's criterion often will be met in symptomatic esophoria. Saladin[7] has recommended a related rule, the 1:1 rule, for use in esophoria.

THE 1:1 RULE

The 1:1 rule states that the base-in recovery should be at least as great as the amount of the esophoria. The base-in recovery value can be taken from the standard Risley rotary prism fusional vergence ranges, or the maximum loose prism power that the patient is capable of fusing can be used for the base-in recovery value. A formula for prism prescription with the 1:1 rule is as follows:

$$\text{base-out prism} = \frac{\text{esophoria} - \text{base-in recovery}}{2}$$

A minus or zero value would indicate that no prism is necessary. If we apply this rule to the case depicted in Figure 6.2, we find that a base-out prism prescription of 2Δ would be recommended:

$$\text{base-out prism} = (\text{esophoria} - \text{base-in recovery})/2$$
$$= (12\Delta - 8\Delta)/2$$
$$= 2\Delta$$

The other treatment alternatives are (1) a plus add for near-point esophoria, which can be derived by the formula for spherical lens power change, or (2) vision training to increase negative fusional convergence so that the base-in recovery equals or exceeds the amount of the esophoria.

REFERENCES

1. Sheard C. Zones of ocular comfort. In: *The Sheard Volume—Selected Writings in Visual and Ophthalmic Optics*. Philadelphia, PA: Chilton; 1957:267–285 (originally published in *Am J Optom*. 1930;7:9–25).
2. Borish I. *Clinical Refraction*. 3rd ed. Boston, MA: Butterworth-Heinemann; 1970:877–879, 900–901.
3. Hofstetter HW. The zone of clear single binocular vision. *Am J Optom Arch Am Acad Optom*. 1945;22:361–384.
4. Sheedy JE, Saladin JJ. Phoria, vergence, and fixation disparity in oculomotor problems. *Am J Optom Physiol Opt*. 1977;54:474–478.
5. Sheedy JE, Saladin JJ. Association of symptoms with measures of oculomotor deficiencies. *Am J Optom Physiol Opt*. 1978;55:670–676.
6. Dalziel CC. Effect of vision training on patients who fail Sheard's criterion. *Am J Optom Physiol Opt*. 1981;58:21–23.
7. Saladin JJ. Horizontal prism prescription. In: Cotter SA, ed. *Clinical Uses of Prism— A Spectrum of Applications—Mosby's Optometric Problem Solving Series*. St Louis, MO: Mosby. 1995:109–147.

SUGGESTED READING

Grisham JD. Treatment of binocular dysfunctions. In: Schor CM, Ciuffreda KJ, eds. *Vergence Eye Movements: Basic and Clinical Aspects*. Boston, MA: Butterworth-Heinemann; 1983:605–646.
Sheedy JE, Saladin JJ. Validity of diagnostic criteria and case analysis in binocular vision disorders. In: Schor CM, Ciuffreda KJ, eds. *Vergence Eye Movements: Basic and Clinical Aspects*. Boston, MA: Butterworth-Heinemann; 1983:517–540.

PRACTICE PROBLEMS

Practice problems for this chapter are given at the end of Chapter 7.

7

Percival's Criterion

Another analytical criterion that can be used in cases of lateral imbalance is Percival's criterion.[1-5] Percival suggested that the positioning of the right- and left-hand boundaries of the zone of clear single binocular vision (ZCSBV) with respect to the demand line is of prime importance. Like Sheard's criterion, Percival's criterion may require separate calculations for different distances, but the criteria differ in that Percival's criterion does not take the phoria into account.

Percival defined a comfort zone, or area of comfort, that occupied the middle third of the width of the ZCSBV and extended from the 0 to the 3.00D stimulus to accommodation level. The comfort zone is illustrated in Figure 7.1. Percival's criterion states that the demand point or orthophoria point for a given test distance should fall within the middle third of the ZCSBV, or, in other words, within the comfort

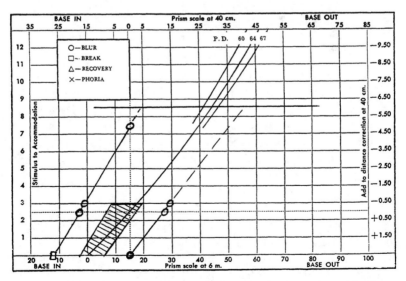

Figure 7.1 Percival's comfort zone for the individual is indicated by the cross-hatched area. Since the demand line falls within the comfort zone, Percival's criterion is met with the subjective refraction. The phoria line is not necessary for determining the comfort zone.

zone. If not, then prism, spherical lens power change, or vision training is called for.

The location of the comfort zone can be determined by either inspection of the graph or computation. If the demand line is outside the comfort zone, Percival's criterion is not met. The computation method requires the following steps. Add the base-in and base-out limits to get the width of the ZCSBV. Then divide this width by 3 to get the width of the comfort zone. If either the base-in or base-out limit is less than the width of the comfort zone, Percival's criterion has not been met.

The easiest way to determine whether Percival's criterion is met is to observe whether the lesser of vergence ranges (base-in or base-out) is at least half of the greater of the vergence ranges. Prism prescription on the basis of Percival's criterion can be achieved by trial and error, inspection of the graph, or formula. In each case, the direction of the base of the prism is toward the greater of the two lateral limits of the ZCSBV.

In the trial-and-error method, various amounts of lateral prism are added to the low (base-in or base-out) limit until it equals or is slightly greater than a third of the total range. The prism prescription is the amount added to the low limit.

In inspection of the graph, the position of the demand point relative to the area of comfort should be noted. The prescribed prism is the distance on the graph in prism diopters from the demand point to the edge of the zone of comfort.

The formula that can be used is

$$P = 1/3G - 2/3L$$

where P represents the prism to be prescribed, G represents the greater of the two lateral limits (base-in or base-out), and L represents the lesser of the two lateral limits (base-in or base-out). If P equals 0 or a minus number, Percival's criterion is met without prism correction.

Once the manipulations have been done, the change in lens power from the subjective refraction that will allow Percival's criterion to be met can be calculated. The formula used for Sheard's criterion is also used here:

$$S = P/A$$

where S represents the spherical lens change, P represents the prism to be prescribed, and A represents the ACA ratio.

To determine the goal of orthoptic vision training as prescribed by Percival's criterion, the greater of the lateral limits (positive relative convergence [PRC] or negative relative convergence [NRC]) is divided by 2. For instance, if the base-in blur is 24 and the base-out blur is 8, then the base-out limit should be increased to 12.

EXAMPLE OF THE USE OF PERCIVAL'S CRITERION

In the situation shown in Figure 7.2, Percival's criterion is met at 6 m but not at 40 cm or 33 cm. For 40 cm

$$P = 1/3G - 2/3L$$
$$= 1/3(26) - 2/3(6)$$
$$= 4\ 2/3\Delta\ \text{base-in}$$

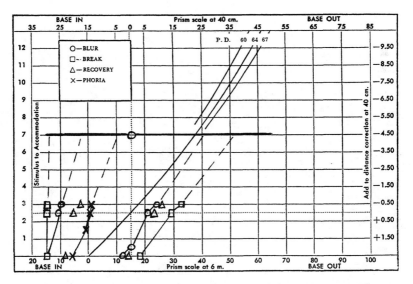

Figure 7.2 The clinical data for the patient in this graph appear in the following table.

	Phoria	Base-in	Base-out	Plus-to-Blur	Minus-to-Blur
6 m	5 exophoria	X/16/8	12/18/14		
40 cm	14 exophoria	26/30/20	6/14/8	+2.00	−4.50
33 cm	17 exophoria	28/33/20	6/12/8		
40 cm − 1.00	16 exophoria				

Amplitude of accommodation, 7.00D.

For 33 cm

$$P = 1/3G - 2/3L$$
$$= 1/3(30) - 2/3(6)$$
$$= 6\Delta \text{ base-in}$$

We can surmise from the graph that the ACA ratio is considerably less than 6. The gradient ACA ratio is $2\Delta/D$ because the amount of exophoria at 40 cm is $\Delta 2$ greater with the $+1.00D$ add.

Since the ACA ratio is low, the spherical lens change will have to be quite large. In this case, from 40 cm we find that

$$S = P/A$$
$$= -4.67/2$$
$$= -2.34 \text{ D}$$

The sign of the spherical lens change will be minus because P is base-in prism. Since such a large lens change is necessary and the amplitude of accommodation is small, this is obviously not a good alternative. In cases of convergence insufficiency, such as this one, base-out vision training is preferred. According to Percival's criterion, the base-out limit (PRC) at 40 cm should be increased to at least 13.

REFERENCES

1. Percival AS. *The Prescribing of Spectacles.* 3rd ed. Bristol, England: John Wright & Sons; 1928:119–136.
2. Borish IM. *Clinical Refraction.* 3rd ed. Boston, MA: Butterworth-Heinemann; 1970:876–877, 899–901.
3. Alpern M. Types of movement. In: Davson H (ed). *Muscular Mechanisms.* 2nd ed. Vol 3 of *The Eye.* New York, NY: Academic; 1969:65–174.
4. Michaels DD. *Visual Optics and Refraction—A Clinical Approach.* 3rd ed. St Louis, MO, Mosby, 1985:381.
5. Robertson KM. Application of Percival's criterion in correcting insignificant hyperopia in a pre-presbyope. *Can J Optom.* 1984;46:39–40.

SUGGESTED READING

Sheedy JE, Saladin JJ. Validity of diagnostic criteria and case analysis in binocular vision disorders. In: Schor CM, Ciuffreda KJ, eds. *Vergence Eye Movements: Basic and Clinical Aspects.* Boston, MA: Butterworth-Heinemann; 1983:517–540.

PRACTICE PROBLEMS

For each of the following patients, answer the questions and graph your findings.

1. What is the width of Percival's comfort zone at 40 cm?

2. What is the demand on fusional convergence at 40 cm?

3. What are the values for the NRC, PRC, negative fusional convergence, and positive functional convergence at 40 cm?

4. What is the reserve at 40 cm?

5. Determine the calculated and gradient ACA ratio.

6. (a) Is Sheard's criterion met at distance? (b) At 40 cm? (c) If not, what prism, lens change, or vision training is required to meet it at these two distances?

7. (a) Is Percival's criterion met at distance? (b) At 40 cm? (c) If not, what prism, lens change, or vision training is required to meet it at these two distances?

8. (a) Is the 1:1 rule met in the cases showing esophoria at distance or at 40 cm? (b) If not, what prism, lens change, or vision training is required to meet it at these distances?

	Patient GH 63-mm PD	Patient JK 64-mm PD	Patient RP 65-mm PD	Patient LP 62-mm PD	Patient MS 60-mm PD
Amplitude of accommodation	5.50D	4.00D	9.00D	8.00D	9.00D
6 m phoria	2 exophoria	4 exophoria	Ortho-phoria		4 esophoria
6 m base-in	X/15/10	X/16/8	X/12/4		X/8/2
6 m base-out	18/22/12	4/8/2	18/30/12		12/22/8
4 m phoria				1 esophoria	
4 m base-in				X/10/4	
4 m base-out				14/24/16	
40 cm phoria	2 exophoria	12 exophoria	5 esophoria	8 exophoria	6 esophoria
40 cm base-in	14/20/12	28/32/20	14/24/6	20/24/8	6/14/3
40 cm base-out	24/28/20	4/12/0	24/34/18	8/16/0	24/32/14
40 cm plus-to-blur	+2.50	+1.25	+2.50	+2.00	+2.25
40 cm minus-to-blur	−2.00	−1.50	−3.00	−5.50	−1.00
40 cm + 1.00 add phoria	5 exophoria		4 exophoria	10 exophoria	1 esophoria
40 cm + 1.00 add base-in	20/24/16		18/24/8	X/24/12	
40 cm + 1.00 add base-out	X/16/8		18/30/12	6/14/2	
33 cm phoria		15 exophoria			
33 cm base-in		28/34/16			
33 cm base-out		12/16/8			

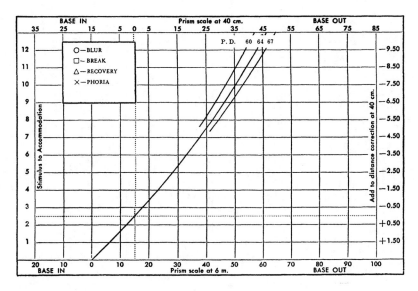

Patient GH

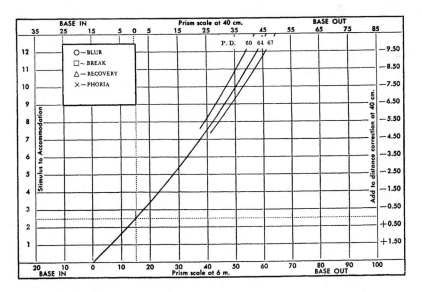

Patient JK

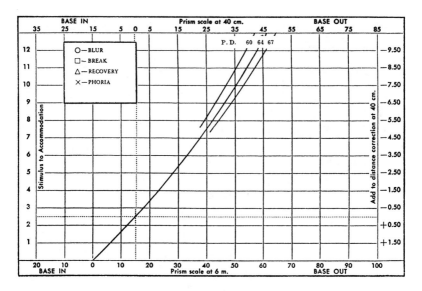

Patient RP

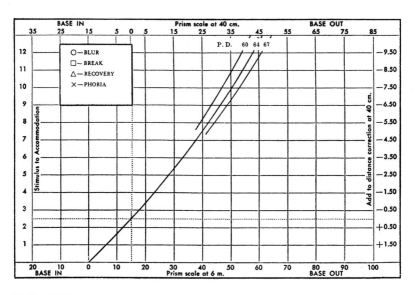

Patient LP

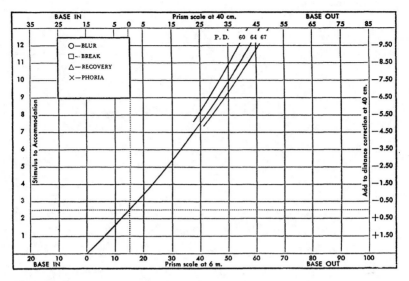

Patient MS

8

Morgan's Norms and Clinical Analysis

Among the many optometrists who have contributed to case analysis is Meredith Morgan.[1-5] This chapter will look at the test norms and the system of clinical analysis that Morgan developed. Although Morgan used a terminology slightly different from ours, his system will be described with the terminology that we have developed.

NORMS

Morgan developed a set of norms from a statistical study of clinical data from a nonselected group of 800 pre-presbyopes. Morgan determined the mean and standard deviation for several findings. He arbitrarily set one-half standard deviation on either side of the mean as his normal range. The values he found are given in Table 8.1. Morgan's mean values are similar to the means reported in other studies.[6-11] The normal ranges derived by Morgan are the most widely used values for the purpose of comparison of individual patient findings to norms.

GROUPS OF TESTS AND THERAPY

Morgan also calculated coefficients of correlation for each test with each of the other tests. In this manner, he could discern relationships between the various tests. On the basis of the magnitudes and signs of the correlation coefficients, he placed each finding in one of three groups, which he labeled A, B, and C (Table 8.2). From the study of graphical analysis, one can readily see why the tests are grouped as they are. For instance, the group A tests fall either on the left-hand side or at the top of the zone of clear single binocular vision (ZCSBV), whereas the group B tests are either on the right-hand side or at the bottom of the ZCSBV. Group C findings are correlated with the slope of the phoria line and the points on the phoria line.

Table 8.1
Mean, standard deviation, and normal values for various clinical tests, as derived by Morgan.

	Mean	Standard Deviation	Normal Range
Distance phoria	1Δ exophoria	2	0 to 2 exophoria
40 cm phoria	3Δ exophoria	5	0 to 6 exophoria
Distance base-in limit			
Blur	X		
Break	7Δ	3	5 to 9
Recovery	4Δ	2	3 to 5
Distance base-out limit			
Blur	9Δ	4	7 to 11
Break	19Δ	8	15 to 23
Recovery	10Δ	4	8 to 12
40 cm base-in limit			
Blur	13Δ	4	11 to 15, or no blur
Break	21Δ	4	19 to 23
Recovery	13Δ	5	10 to 16
40 cm base-out limit			
Blur	17Δ	5	14 to 20, or no blur
Break	21Δ	6	18 to 24
Recovery	11Δ	7	7 to 15
40 cm plus-to-blur	+2.00D	0.50	+1.75 to +2.25
40 cm minus-to-blur	−2.37D	1.12	−1.75 to −3.00
Gradient ACA ratio	4Δ/D	2	3 to 5
Amplitude of accommodation	16.0 − (0.25)(age)	2.00	16.0 − (0.25)(age) ±1.00

Most patients fit into one of three categories: (1) group A and group B findings normal, (2) group A findings low and group B findings high, or (3) group A findings high and group B findings low. Morgan suggests that when a symptomatic individual exhibits low group A findings, the therapy options are plus sphere adds, base-out prism, or vision training. When asthenopia is accompanied by low group B findings, the treatments available are minus sphere adds, base-in prism, or vision training. Which method is applied, Morgan further proposed, depends on the results of the group C tests, the age of the patient, and professional judgment. A clinical analysis system based on comparisons to norms is sometimes referred to as "normative analysis." Morgan's system of analysis could thus be considered a form of normative analysis. Morgan did emphasize, however, that caution should be exercised in comparing an isolated finding to its norm ("interpatient comparison"). Different test

Table 8.2
Grouping of tests suggested by Morgan.

Group A
  40 cm base-in blur, break, and recovery
  40 cm minus-to-blur
  Amplitude of accommodation
  6 m base-in break and recovery

Group B
  40 cm base-out blur, break, and recovery
  40 cm plus-to-blur
  6 m base-out blur, break, and recovery

Group C
  Gradient ACA ratio
  6 m phoria
  40 cm phoria
  Calculated ACA ratio

---

findings for an individual patient also should be compared with each other. A graphical display of accommodation and convergence data, like that discussed in previous chapters, provides a tool for such intrapatient comparisons.

REFERENCES

1. Morgan MW. The clinical aspects of accommodation and convergence. *Am J Optom Arch Am Acad Optom.* 1944;21:301–313.
2. Morgan MW. Analysis of clinical data. *Am J Optom Arch Am Acad Optom.* 1944;21:477–491.
3. Morgan MW. The analysis of clinical data. *Optom Weekly.* 1964;55:27–34; 55:23–25.
4. Morgan MW. Accommodation and vergence. *Am J Optom Arch Am Acad Optom.* 1968;45:417–454.
5. Morgan MW. The Maddox analysis of vergence. In: Schor CM, Ciuffreda KJ, eds. *Vergence Eye Movements: Basic and Clinical Aspects.* Boston, MA: Butterworth-Heinemann; 1983:15–21.
6. Haines HF. Normal values of visual functions and their application in case analysis. Part IV. The analysis of findings and determination of normals. *Am J Optom Arch Am Acad Optom.* 1941;18:58–73.
7. Haines HF. Normal values of visual functions and their application in case analysis. Part V. Presenting a table of normal values for visual functions. *Am J Optom Arch Am Acad Optom.* 1941;10:112–116.
8. Betts EA, Austin AS. Seeing problems of school children. *Optom Weekly.* 1941; 32:369–371.

9. Shepard CF. The most probable "expecteds." *Optom Weekly.* 1941;32:530–541.

10. Saladin JJ, Sheedy JE. Population study of fixation disparity, heterophoria, and vergence. *Am J Optom Physiol Opt.* 1970;55:744–750.

11. Jackson TW, Goss DA. Variation and correlation of standard clinical phoropter tests of phorias, vergence ranges, and relative accommodation in a sample of school-age children. *J Am Optom Assoc.* 1991;62:540–547.

SUGGESTED READING

Borish IM. *Clinical Refraction.* 3rd ed. Boston, MA: Butterworth-Heinemann; 1970:900–923.

Michaels DD. *Visual Optics and Refraction—A Clinical Approach.* 3rd ed. St Louis, MO: Mosby, 1985:378–380.

Morgan MW. The analysis of clinical data. *Optom Weekly.* 1964;55:27–34, 55:23–25.

PRACTICE PROBLEMS

1. Graph Morgan's norms. Keep the appearance of the following graph in mind as an example of a normal set findings.

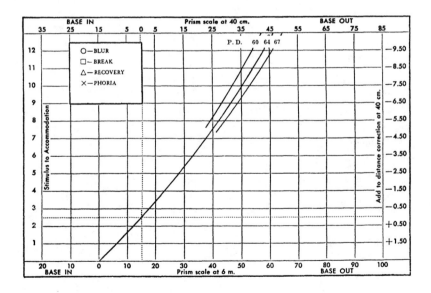

2. What is the calculated ACA ratio using Morgan's mean phorias? Compare this with the mean gradient ACA ratio, and if different, explain why.

3. Which is the greater at 40 cm, the positive width or the negative width of the ZCSBV, based on Morgan's means?

4. Which shows more variability: (a) distance or near-point phorias? (b) Base-in or base-out fusional amplitudes?

9

Introduction to Fixation Disparity

Fixation disparity is a condition in which the images of a binocularly fixated object do not stimulate exactly corresponding retinal points but still fall within Panum's fusional areas, the object thus being seen singly.[1] The existence of fixation disparity indicates that there is a slight overconvergence (eso fixation disparity) or underconvergence (exo fixation disparity) of the lines of sight under binocular condition. This misalignment is very small, since sensory fusion would not otherwise be possible. Fixation disparity usually is measured in minutes of arc. If it were expressed in prism diopters, it usually would be less than 0.25Δ and almost always would be less than 0.75Δ.[2]

Fixation disparity usually is measured by subjective alignment of two small lines or bars, one seen by each eye. Other than the marks used for alignment, all features of the test target are seen binocularly. The amount of fixation disparity is the sum of the angular eccentricities of the subjectively aligned marks with respect to the convergence stimulus value of the binocularly fused components of the test target (Figure 9.1).

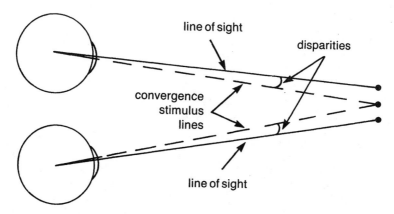

Figure 9.1 Exo fixation disparity. The angle of disparity is the sum of the angular disparities of the two eyes. If one eye is fixating precisely, all of the disparity will be represented in the angular deviation of the other eye.

Examples of devices that can be used to measure fixation disparity are the Wesson Fixation Disparity Card[3] and the Sheedy Disparometer.[4] For example, in the Disparometer, there are several pairs of marks with different preset separations; the pairs can be shown separately until one with apparent alignment is picked. For illustration, a schematic of the Disparometer is shown in Figure 9.2.

The amount of fixation disparity measured is a function of individual characteristics of patients and testing conditions. Of the latter, the most important features are (1) the size of the area in which binocular vision is excluded, (2) the amount of fusional convergence required, and (3)

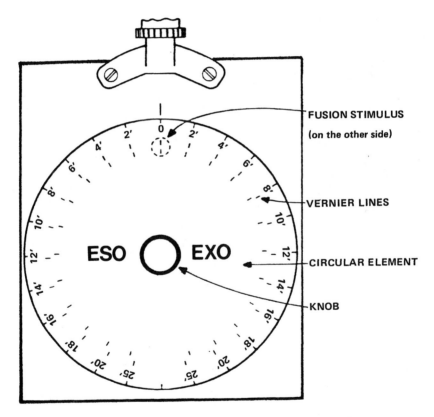

Figure 9.2 A schematic diagram of the Sheedy Disparometer. The illustrated pairs of marks are shown to the patient one at a time in the circular window until a pair that subjectively appears aligned is chosen. The examiner can then read the actual physical separation of the lines from a window at the back of the instrument. The physical separation of the pair of lines that appears perfectly aligned is a measure of the fixation disparity.

(Reprinted with permission from Sheedy JE. Fixation disparity analysis of oculomotor imbalance. *Am J Optom Physiol Opt.* 1980;57:632–639.)

the length of time allowed for adaptation to the prisms in effect while or before the fixation disparity is measured.[5-8] The larger the area without fusion clues, the greater the fixation disparity. As the amount of positive fusional convergence increases, fixation disparity shifts in the exo direction. This indicates an increasing underconvergence as the level of convergence increases. As the amount of negative fusional convergence required for single vision increases, fixation disparity moves in the eso direction. Therefore, as base-in or base-out prism power is increased, fixation disparity becomes more eso or exo, respectively. As the time allowed for adaptation to the prism is increased, fixation disparity decreases.

Stress associated with the use of fusional convergence can result in asthenopia. Clinical fixation disparity measurement is a useful diagnostic tool because it is related to fusional convergence effort.[7-9] This is easily demonstrated by the observation that fixation disparity varies as a function of the prism power through which a patient views. In addition, there is a correlation of fixation disparity with dissociated phoria[10-12] (Figure 9.3).

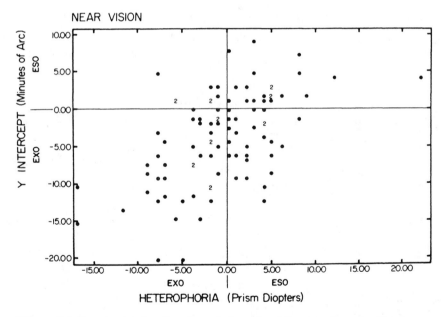

Figure 9.3 Scatterplot showing the relationship of fixation disparity (fixation disparity curve [FDC] y-intercept) with dissociated phoria. Fixation disparity in minutes of arc is plotted on the y-axis, and dissociated phoria in prism diopters is plotted on the x-axis. Each point represents findings for one individual.

(Reprinted with permission from Saladin JJ, Sheedy JE. Population study of fixation disparity, heterophoria, and vergence. *Am J Optom Physiol Opt.* 1978; 55:744–50.)

ASSOCIATED PHORIA

Many of the clinical fixation disparity devices cannot actually measure fixation disparity; instead they detect the presence of a fixation disparity and allow the examiner to determine the prism power that reduces fixation disparity to 0. These instruments are characterized by the monocularly viewed marks being physically aligned and not movable with respect to each other. A fixation disparity exists when the patient reports that the marks or bars are not perfectly aligned perceptually. Typically, the top vertical bar is seen by the right eye and the bottom is seen by the left eye. Thus, if the patient reports the top line being to the right of the bottom line, an eso fixation disparity exists; if the top line is to the left of the bottom one, an exo fixation disparity exists. The amount of base-in prism required to reduce an exo disparity to 0 or the amount of base-out prism required to reduce an eso fixation disparity to 0 is referred to as the "associated phoria."

To avoid confusion, we should distinguish between dissociated and associated phorias. Prior to this chapter, we were examining dissociated phorias. "Dissociated" refers to the fact that the eyes are dissociated; that is, binocular vision is not allowed in any part of the visual field, except, perhaps unavoidably, in the extreme peripheral portions of it. The nonfused condition of dissociated phoria testing is achieved basically by four categories of methods: (1) exclusion, such as the cover test; (2) diplopia or displacement, such as the von Graefe technique; (3) distortion, such as the Maddox rod; and (4) nonfusable or independent objects, such as those present on stereoscopic phoria cards. On an associated phoria measurement, binocular vision is present throughout the visual field except for a small area surrounding the two monocularly viewed fiducial marks.

Usually, the amount of an associated phoria is less than the corresponding dissociated phoria in a given individual. Associated phorias and dissociated phorias are fairly highly correlated,[10–12] but some individuals yield prism values with opposite prism base orientations on the two tests. This occurrence, referred to as "paradoxical fixation disparity," is most commonly found in patients who have received orthoptics to increase fusional vergence amplitudes. The typical paradoxical fixation disparity patient shows an exo dissociated phoria with an eso fixation disparity.[8,13] The relationship of dissociated phoria and associated phoria is illustrated in Figure 9.4.

THE FIXATION DISPARITY CURVE AND ITS PARAMETERS

An FDC is a plot of the amount of fixation disparity (y- axis) obtained through various amounts of prism (x-axis). The curves for different pa-

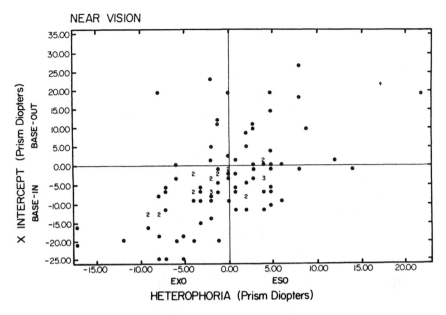

Figure 9.4 Scatterplot showing the relationship of associated phoria (FDC x-intercept) with dissociated phoria. The FDC x-intercept (associated phoria) in prism diopters is represented on the y-axis of this scatterplot. The x-axis of this scatterplot shows dissociated phoria measurements in prism diopters.

(Reprinted with permission from Saladin JJ, Sheedy JE. Population study of fixation disparity, heterophoria, and vergence. *Am J Optom Physiol Opt.* 1978;55:744–750.)

tients vary in their configuration, vertical placement, and lateral placement. Their configurations are divided into four categories, called "curve types" (Figure 9.5), by Ogle et al.[10] Type I has a sigmoid curve shape with a steep rise in fixation disparity near both the base-in and base-out fusional limits. Approximately 60% of individuals have type I curves. Type II and type III curves have flat segments on the base-out and base-in sides, respectively. The prevalence of these types of curves is approximately 25% for Type II and 10% for type III.[14] The configuration of FDCs is related to prism adaptation. Prism adaptation also is known as "vergence adaptation" or "fusional aftereffects."[8,15–18] Prism adaptation often is viewed as a shift in the tonic convergence level after the use of fusional convergence. One way that it is demonstrated is to measure dissociated phorias before and after viewing through prism for some period of time. Viewing through base-out prism results in a shift of the phoria toward eso, and viewing through base-in will cause the phoria to shift in the exo direction. Prism adaptation varies from one patient to another. Schor[8,13] has found that prism adaptation and fixation disparity are inversely related and that persons with type II or III curves have asymmetric prism adaptation for convergent and divergent stimuli. Cases of greater base-

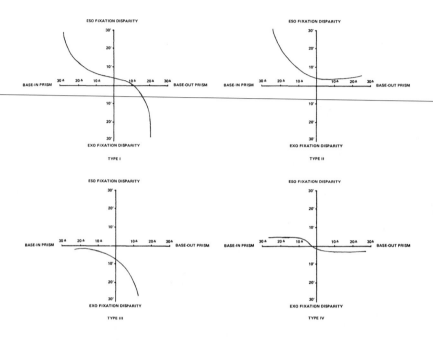

Figure 9.5 The four types of fixation disparity curves.

(Reprinted by permission from Sheedy JE. Fixation disparity analysis of oculomotor imbalance. *Am J Optom Physiol Opt.* 1980;57:632–639.)

out prism adaptation correspond to type II curves, and cases of greater base-in prism adaptation are found with type III curves. The type IV curve shows changes in fixation disparity with prism in the central portion of the curve and little or no change toward the fusional limits on both sides. The prevalence of type IV curves is approximately 5%.[14] A type IV curve may indicate a deficiency of sensory or motor fusion.[7,8]

Other important parameters of an FDC are its slope, y-intercept, x-intercept, and center of symmetry. The slope is commonly derived using a best-fitting straight line through points in a range of approximately 3Δ base-in to 3Δ base-out.[12,19] The y-intercept is the amount of fixation disparity with 0 prism. The x-intercept is the amount of prism that reduces the fixation disparity to 0. Thus, the x-intercept point on the curve is the associated phoria. The center of symmetry is the flattest central region of the FDC. In other words, the center of symmetry is the point on the curve where the slope is closest to zero. If the FDC has a portion that is horizontal (zero slope), then the center of symmetry is the point on the flat segment of the curve where the prism power is the least.

All the parameters of an FDC are illustrated in Figure 9.6. The ends of the curves generally correspond to points of diplopia, and thus the x-axis values at the ends of the curves should be similar to the negative relative convergence and positive relative convergence findings.

THE CHANGE IN FIXATION DISPARITY WITH LENSES

We can vary the relative amounts of accommodative and fusional convergence exerted under binocular conditions by placing lenses of various powers before the eyes. Since fixation disparity is related to the amount of fusional convergence being used, it will vary with lens power and sign. Plus lenses, by decreasing accommodative convergence, will increase the required positive fusional convergence for convergent stim-

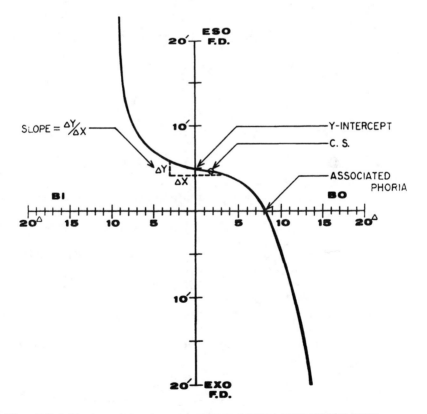

Figure 9.6 Fixation disparity parameters in a type 1 FDC. Besides curve type, the major parameters of an FDC are slope, y-intercept, x-intercept (associated phoria), and center of symmetry.

uli and will decrease the required negative fusional convergence for divergent stimuli. Plus lenses will thus shift the FDC down and to the left. By the opposite effect on accommodative convergence, minus lenses will shift the curve up and to the right. An eso fixation disparity can thus be reduced to 0 with plus lenses, and an exo fixation disparity can be reduced to 0 with minus lenses.

REFERENCES

1. Cline D, Hofstetter HW, Griffin JR. *Dictionary of Visual Science.* 4th ed. Radnor, PA: Chilton; 1989:205.
2. Sheedy JE. Actual measurement of fixation disparity and its use in diagnosis and treatment. *J Am Optom Assoc.* 1980;51:1079–1084.
3. Wesson MD, Koenig R. A new clinical method for direct measurement of fixation disparity. *South J Optom.* 1983;1:48–52.
4. Sheedy JE. Fixation disparity analysis of oculomotor imbalance. *Am J Optom Physiol Opt.* 1980;57:632–639.
5. Ogle KN, Mussey F, Prangen A deH. Fixation disparity and the fusional processes in binocular single vision. *Am J Ophthalmol.* 1949;32:1069–1087.
6. Carter DB. Fixation disparity with and without foveal fusion contours. *Am J Optom Arch Am Acad Optom.* 1964;41:729–736.
7. Carter DB. Parameters of fixation disparity. *Am J Optom Physiol Opt.* 1980; 57:610–617.
8. Schor CM. Fixation disparity and vergence adaptation. In: Schor CM, Ciuffreda KJ, eds. *Vergence Eye Movements: Basic and Clinical Aspects.* Boston, MA: Butterworth-Heinemann; 1983:465–516.
9. Ogle KN. *Researches in Binocular Vision.* New York, NY: Hafner; 1950:69–93.
10. Ogle KN, Martens TG, Dyer JA. *Oculomotor Imbalance in Binocular Vision and Fixation Disparity.* Philadelphia, PA: Lea & Febiger; 1967:75–119.
11. McCullough RW. The fixation disparity-heterophoria relationship. *J Am Optom Assoc.* 1978;49:369–372.
12. Saladin JJ, Sheedy JE. Population study of fixation disparity, heterophoria, and vergence. *Am J Optom Physiol Opt.* 1970;55:744–750.
13. Schor GM. Fixation disparity: a steady state error of disparity-induced vergence. *Am J Optom Physiol Opt.* 1980;57:618–631.
14. Sheedy JE, Saladin JJ. Validity of diagnostic criteria and case analysis in binocular vision disorders. In: Schor CM, Ciuffreda KJ, eds. *Vergence Eye Movements: Basic and Clinical Aspects.* Boston, MA: Butterworth-Heinemann; 1983: 517–540.
15. Carter DB. Effects of prolonged wearing of prism. *Am J Optom Arch Am Acad Optom.* 1963;40:265–273.
16. Carter DB. Fixation disparity and heterophoria following prolonged wearing of prism. *Am J Optom Arch Am Acad Optom.* 1965;42:141–152.
17. Alpern M. Types of movement. In: Davson H, ed. *Muscular Mechanisms.* 2nd ed. Vol 3 of *The Eye.* New York, NY: Academic; 1969:65–174.
18. Henson DB, North R. Adaptation to prism-induced heterophoria. *Am J Optom Physiol Opt.* 1980;57:129–137.

19. Wick BC. Horizontal deviations. In: Amos JF, ed. *Diagnosis and Management in Vision Care*. Boston, MA: Butterworth-Heinemann; 1987:461–510.

SUGGESTED READING

Carter DB. Parameters of fixation disparity. *Am J Optom Physiol Opt*. 1980;57: 610–617.

Goss DA. Fixation disparity. In: Eskridge JB, Amos JF, Bartlett JD, eds. *Clinical Procedures in Optometry*. Philadelphia, PA: Lippincott; 1991:716–726.

Ogle KN, Martens TG, Dyer JA. *Oculomotor Imbalance in Binocular Vision and Fixation Disparity*. Philadelphia, PA: Lea & Febiger; 1967.

Reading RW. *Binocular Vision: Foundations and Applications*. Boston, MA: Butterworth-Heinemann; 1983:131–149.

PRACTICE PROBLEMS

1. List and describe the five main parameters of FDCs.

2. In Figure 9.5, label the associated phoria on each of the curves.

3. Which test condition factors have significant effects on the amount of fixation disparity?

10

Clinical Use of Fixation Disparity

Some clinicians feel that a complete work-up of vergence disorders includes both analysis of dissociated phorias and fusional vergence findings and analysis of fixation disparity. Because the testing conditions and the variables measured are different, analysis of fixation disparity and analysis of dissociated phorias and fusional amplitudes do not completely substitute for each other. For instance, Schor[1] has stated that when an oculomotor imbalance has been confirmed by dissociated phorias and fusional amplitudes in a symptomatic patient, a prism prescription can be effectively derived from fixation disparity data. It also is possible for an individual without a significant dissociated phoria to have a fixation disparity.

In two studies of the relationship between asthenopia and various clinical criteria of lateral imbalances, Sheedy and Saladin[2,3] confirmed the overall utility of Sheard's criterion. However, other measures, such as the amount of the dissociated phoria and certain fixation disparity variables, were better discriminators of asthenopia in esophoria. To restate, it is helpful to supplement dissociated phoria-fusional amplitude analysis with fixation disparity analysis in esophoria. Other work by Sheedy and Saladin[4,5] suggests that this also is true of the high exophoria often induced by presbyopic adds.

Sheedy and Saladin[2,3] also showed that the diagnostic value of fixation disparity is maximized by the use of the entire fixation disparity curve (FDC). Whether one is able to determine the entire FDC or just the associated phoria depends on the available instrumentation. The instrumentation and methods for measurement and interpretation of associated phorias and fixation disparity are discussed below.

MEASUREMENT OF ASSOCIATED PHORIAS

Instrumentation for the measurement of distance-associated phorias includes the American Optical (AO) vectographic slide, the Bernell lantern far-point target, and the Mallett far-point testing unit (Figures 10.1, 10.2, and 10.3, respectively).[6–9] The AO vectographic slide is de-

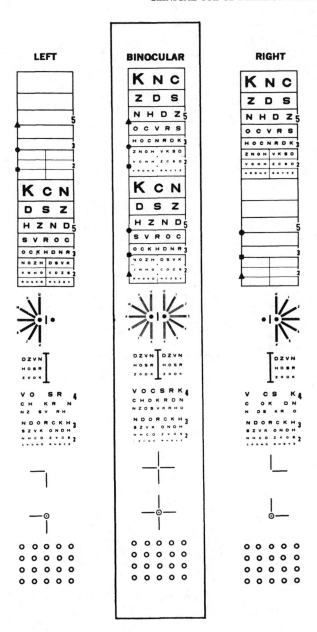

Figure 10.1 The AO vectographic slide. Some portions of the chart are seen with the right eye and some with the left eye, as indicated in the diagram. On the associated phoria target the upper vertical line and the horizontal line on the right are seen with the right eye, and the other two lines are seen with the left eye.

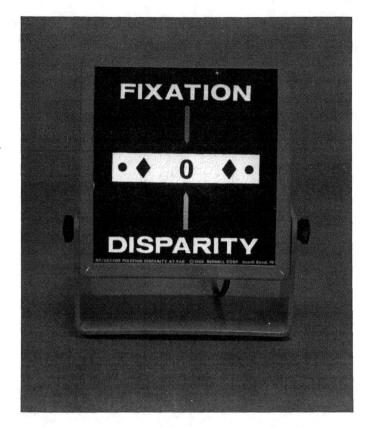

Figure 10.2 The Bernell lantern far-point-associated phoria target. The upper line is seen with the right eye.

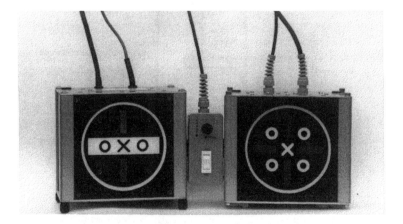

Figure 10.3 Mallett units for distance-associated phoria measurement. On the left is the distance Mallett unit introduced in the 1960s by Mallett that has been widely used since. On the right is the distance Mallett unit now being manufactured. The red lines used for associated phoria measurement, difficult to see in this black and white photograph, are just above and below the X on each instrument, as well as to either side of the X on the new Mallett unit.

signed for use in the AO projector. The Bernell test lantern usually is placed on a table, and the Mallett unit for far-point testing can be placed on a table or mounted on a wall.

Instruments that can be used to measure near-associated phorias include the Bernell lantern near-point target, the Mallett near-point units, and the Borish card (Figures 10.4, 10.5, 10.6, and 10.7).[6-10] The Bernell test lantern has a near-point slide that can be alternated with the far-point-associated phoria slide. As noted above, it usually is used on a table, but can be hand-held for near-point testing. One Mallett near-point unit is hand-held or placed on a table. The other Mallett near-point unit is designed to be placed on a reading rod. The Borish card can be hand-held or placed on a phoropter reading rod.

For use of each of these devices the patient must view through polaroid filter test goggles or the polaroid filter setting in the phoropter. The vertical lines are used for the measurement of the horizontal-associated phoria. The upper line is seen by the right eye, and the lower line is seen by the left eye. Most of the other features in the targets are seen by both eyes, and thus serve as "fusion locks." The examiner asks the patient whether the top line is directly above or to the right or left of the lower line. If it is directly above the lower line the associated phoria is zero. If the top line is to the left of the bottom line, an exo fixation disparity exists and the minimum amount of base-in prism that aligns the two vertical lines is the associated phoria. If the top line is to the right, the associated phoria is the amount of base-out prism that neutralizes the eso fixation disparity.

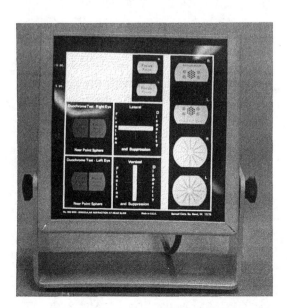

Figure 10.4
Near-point slide for the Bernell lantern. The associated phoria targets are in the middle (lateral associated phoria) and in the lower center (vertical associated phoria) of the slide.

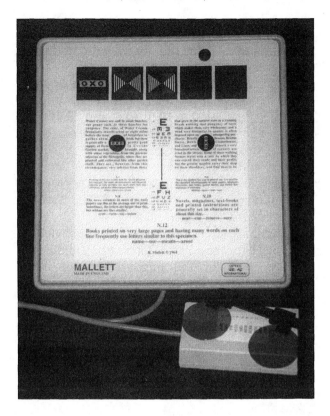

Figure 10.5 A Mallett unit for near-point testing. This
unit is designed to be hand-held or placed on a table.
The associated phoria targets are in the circular windows
within the areas of reading text and on the upper left
portion of the unit.

Distance-associated phoria measurements taken with the AO vectographic slide agree well with those measured with the distance Mallett
unit.[8] Associated phorias at near using the Borish card are similar to
those obtained with the near-point Bernell unit[8] and with the near-point
Mallett unit.[11]

PRESCRIPTION FROM ASSOCIATED PHORIAS

Mallett[6,7] introduced the idea that the existence of fixation disparity
indicates that fusional convergence has not adequately compensated for
a heterophoria. Thus, an individual with an uncompensated phoria is
one who has dissociated and associated phorias with the same prism
base orientations. Using this concept, Mallett recommended some

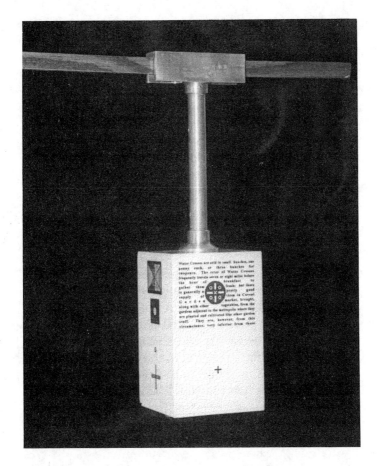

Figure 10.6 A Mallett unit for near-point testing. This unit is designed to be placed on a phoropter reading rod. The associated phoria target is in the circular area on the side of the instrument containing the paragraph of reading text.

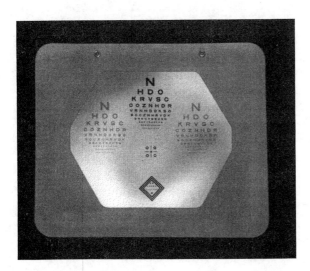

Figure 10.7
One side of the Borish near-point chart. The vertical and horizontal lines for lateral- and vertical-associated phoria measurements, respectively, are in the middle of the card.

prescription guidelines. For the young uncompensated exophore, base-out vision training or the minus add that reduces fixation disparity to 0 should be given. For the older uncompensated exophore, the base-in prism indicated by the associated phoria should be prescribed. In a patient with uncompensated esophoria at distance, the treatment of choice is the base-out prism of the associated phoria, and for the near-point uncompensated esophore, the plus add that eliminates the fixation disparity or a combination of a plus add and base-out prism can be used.

DETERMINATION OF FIXATION DISPARITY CURVES

Devices for the measurement of associated phorias indicate whether the lines of sight of the two eyes are aligned, but they do not indicate the amount of misalignment of the lines of sight; the prism added to achieve alignment is then the associated phoria. In contrast, when we measure fixation disparity we are measuring the amount of misalignment of the lines of sight with respect to the convergence stimulus presented by the target distance. Instruments that allow a measurement of fixation disparity at near-point include the Sheedy Disparometer (Figures 10.8 and 10.9) and the Wesson fixation disparity card (Figure 10.10).[8,9,12–14].

Polaroid testing goggles or the polaroid filter phoropter setting is necessary for the use of either the Sheedy Disparometer or the Wesson fixation disparity card. When using the Sheedy Disparometer, the examiner rotates pairs of vertical lines (see Figure 9.2) through the window visible to the patient (see Figure 10.8). The patient reports when the top line is directly above the bottom line. The amount of misalignment indicated on the back of the Disparometer (see Figure 10.9) provides a measure of the amount of fixation disparity in minutes of arc. Testing with the Wesson fixation disparity card involves asking the patient to which of the upper lines the arrow is pointing (see Figure 10.10). The examiner can then refer to the table in the upper right corner of the card to note the amount of the fixation disparity. Both devices can either be hand-held or mounted on the phoropter reading rod.

To plot an FDC, fixation disparity is measured at several different prism settings. Prism power can be set by the phoropter rotary prism or by placing loose prisms in a trial frame.[15] Sheedy[13] has recommended measuring fixation disparity with zero prism, then with base-in prism, increasing the power in 3 increments to diplopia, and then with base-out prism in 3 increments to diplopia. Wick[16] prefers to alternate base-in and base-out prism in the following order: 0, 3Δ base-in, 3Δ base-out, 6Δ base-in, 6Δ base-out, 9Δ base-in, 9Δ base-out, etc., to diplopia with

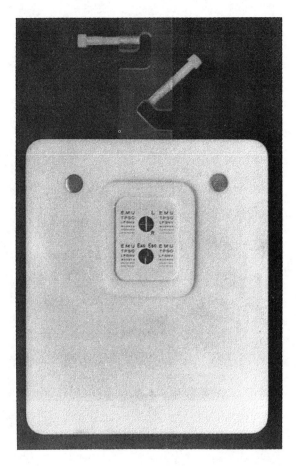

Figure 10.8
Patient's side of the
Sheedy Disparometer.
Pairs of lines are rotated
through the round win-
dows until the patient reports that they are aligned.
Pairs of vertical lines for
lateral fixation disparity
are visible in the lower
window. The upper win-
dow contains targets for
vertical fixation disparity.

both base-in and base-out. Using the latter order, if diplopia occurs much earlier on one prism base direction than on the other, alternation can be continued with the use of a prism power that can just be fused on the side with the lower fusional range; this may serve to limit an effect of increasing prism adaptation on the shape of the curve.[17]

The x-axis on an FDC is the amount of prism in prism diopters. Base-in is to the left on the x-axis. Base-out increases to the right on the graph because greater base-out represents a greater convergence stimulus. The amount of the fixation disparity in minutes of arc is plotted on the y-axis. Eso fixation disparity (the eyes slightly convergent with respect to the convergence stimulus) is above the x-axis. Exo fixation disparity (slight divergence of the lines of sight with respect to the target) is below the x-axis. An example is shown in Figure 10.11.

The parameters of the FDC (curve type, slope, y-intercept, x-intercept, and center of symmetry) were defined in Chapter 9. Since the x-intercept is the point where fixation disparity is equal to zero, the

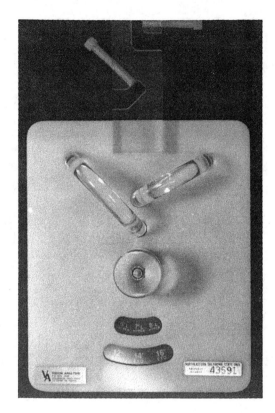

Figure 10.9
Examiner's side of the Sheedy Disparometer. The separations of the target lines are changed using the knob in the center until the patient reports alignment. The amount of fixation disparity is then read from the center of the display at the bottom of the instrument.

x-value (prism setting) at that point is the associated phoria. However, it should be kept in mind that FDC x-intercepts usually are greater in magnitude than the associated phorias measured with the near-point Bernell target, the Borish card, or the Mallett near-point unit.[8,18]

The FDC in Figure 10.11 is a type I curve. The slope from 3Δ base-in to 3Δ base-out is −0.67 minutes of arc per prism diopter. The y-intercept is 2 minutes of arc exo, and the x-intercept is 3Δ base-in. The center of symmetry is at zero prism.

PRESCRIPTION FROM FIXATION DISPARITY CURVES

The guidelines for prescribing from FDCs are summarized from Sheedy,[12,13] Sheedy and Saladin,[19] Schor,[20] and Wick.[16] Curve type may be the best diagnostic parameter of the FDC. Persons with type I curves usually are asymptomatic; those with types II, III, and IV curves are commonly symptomatic. The type I FDC patient who does have asthenopia usually has an FDC with a high slope and is managed well with vision

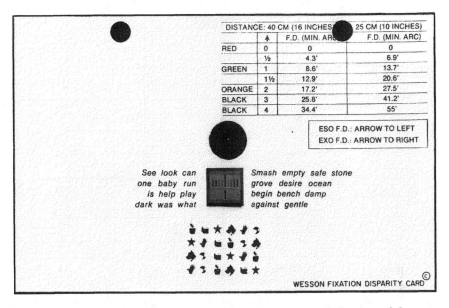

Figure 10.10 Wesson fixation disparity card. The arrow at the bottom of the polarized area in the center of the card is seen by the left eye when the patient wears the appropriate polaroid goggles. The lines above the arrow are seen by the right eye. The patient reports to which line the arrow appears to be pointing. Each of the marks represents a particular amount of fixation disparity calibrated for test distances of 25 and 40 cm as shown in the upper right corner of the card.

training. A successful vision training program is correlated with a flattening of the FDC slope.

Most type II FDCs occur in patients with esophoria. Patients with type II curves respond better to prism prescription and plus lens adds than to vision training. Type III curves usually are associated with high exophoria. Patients with type III curves can be managed with prism prescription or vision training, although vision training is less likely to be successful' than in type I curve patients. Prism prescriptions for types II and III curve patients should be the amount of prism that allows the patient to function at the flat portion of the curve. In other words, the prism power at the center of symmetry should be prescribed.

There is no general agreement among clinicians whether prism or vision training is preferable for patients with type IV curves. A type IV curve may indicate poor sensory or motor fusion, or both.

Patients with steeper FDC slopes are more likely to be symptomatic. Flatter slopes are correlated with higher levels of prism adaptation.[21] A high value for the y-intercept also can be a sign of an oculomotor problem. Slope and y-intercept can be useful for diagnostic and management

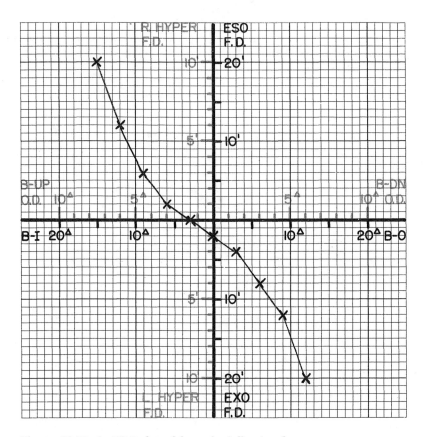

Figure 10.11 An FDC plotted from the following data:

Prism Setting (in Prism Diopters)	Fixation Disparity (in Minutes of Arc)
0	2 exo
3 base-in	0
3 base-out	4 exo
6 base-in	2 eso
6 base-out	8 exo
9 base-in	6 eso
9 base-out	12 exo
12 base-in	12 eso
12 base-out	20 exo
15 base-in	20 eso
15 base-out	diplopia
18 base-in	diplopia

decision making, but they do not directly yield a numerical value for lens or prism prescription.

Some patients complain of instability of the nonius lines during fixation disparity testing. This can result in an irregularly shaped FDC. An irregular FDC can be an indication of an accommodation problem. If so, vision training to improve accommodation will result in a smoothing of the FDC.

REFERENCES

1. Schor CM. Fixation disparity: a steady state error. *Am J Optom Physiol Opt.* 1980;57:618–631.
2. Sheedy JE, Saladin JJ. Phoria, vergence, and fixation disparity in oculomotor problems. *Am J Optom Physiol Opt.* 1977;54:474–478.
3. Sheedy JE, Saladin JJ. Association of symptoms with measures of oculomotor deficiencies. *Am J Optom Physiol Opt.* 1978;55:670– 676.
4. Sheedy JE, Saladin JJ. Exophoria at near in presbyopia. *Am J Optom Physiol Opt.* 1975;52:474–481.
5. Sheedy JE. Analysis of oculomotor balance. *Rev Optom.* 1979;116:44–45.
6. Mallett RFJ. Fixation disparity in clinical practice. *Aust J Optom.* 1969;52: 97–109.
7. Mallett RFJ. Fixation disparity-its genesis in relation to asthenopia. *Ophthalmic Optician.* 1974;14:1159–1168.
8. Brownlee GA, Goss DA. Comparisons of commercially available devices for the measurement of fixation disparity and associated phorias. *J Am Optom Assoc.* 1988;59:451–460.
9. Goss DA. Fixation disparity. In: Eskridge JB, Amos JF, Bartlett JD, eds. *Clinical Procedures in Optometry.* Philadelphia, PA: Lippincott; 1991:716–726.
10. Borish IM. The Borish nearpoint chart. *J Am Optom Assoc.* 1978;49:41–44.
11. Yee L. Comparison of nearpoint techniques. *J Am Optom Assoc.* 1981;52: 579–582.
12. Sheedy JE. Fixation disparity analysis of oculomotor imbalance. *Am J Optom Physiol Opt.* 1980;57:632–639.
13. Sheedy JE. Actual measurement of fixation disparity and its use in diagnosis and treatment. *J Am Optom Assoc.* 1980;51:1079–1084.
14. Wesson MD, Koenig R. A new clinical method for direct measurement of fixation disparity. *South J Optom.* 1983;1:48–52.
15. Frantz KA, Scharre JE. Comparison of Disparometer fixation disparity curves as measured with and without the phoropter. *Optom Vis Sci.* 1990;67:117–122.
16. Wick BC. Horizontal deviations. In: Amos JF, ed. *Diagnosis and Management in Vision Care.* Boston, MA: Butterworth-Heinemann; 1987:461–510.
17. Scheiman M, Wick B. *Clinical Management of Binocular Vision-Heterophoric, Accommodative, and Eye Movement Disorders.* Philadelphia, PA: Lippincott; 1994: 450–451.
18. Wildsoet CF, Cameron KD. The effect of illumination and foveal fusion lock on clinical fixation disparity measurements with the Sheedy Disparometer. *Ophthal Physiol Opt.* 1985;5:171–178.

19. Sheedy JE, Saladin JJ. Validity of diagnostic criteria and case analysis in binocular vision disorders. In: Schor CM, Ciuffreda KJ, eds. *Vergence Eye Movements: Basic and Clinical Aspects.* Boston, MA: Butterworth-Heinemann; 1983: 517–540.
20. Schor CM. Fixation disparity and vergence adaptation. In: Schor CM, Ciuffreda KJ, eds. *Vergence Eye Movements: Basic and Clinical Aspects.* Boston, MA: Butterworth-Heinemann; 1983:465–516.
21. Schor CM. The influence of rapid prism adaptation upon fixation disparity. *Vision Res.* 1979;19:757–765.

SUGGESTED READING

Goss DA. Fixation disparity. In: Eskridge JB, Amos JF, Bartlett JD, eds. *Clinical Procedures in Optometry.* Philadelphia, PA: Lippincott; 1991:716–726.
Schor CM. Fixation disparity and vergence adaptation. In: Schor CM, Ciuffreda KJ, eds. *Vergence Eye Movements: Basic and Clinical Aspects.* Boston, MA: Butterworth-Heinemann; 1983:465–516.
Sheedy JE. Actual measurement of fixation disparity and its use in diagnosis and treatment. *J Am Optom Assoc.* 1980;51:1079–1084.

PRACTICE PROBLEMS

1. List the instruments that can be used to measure associated phorias and those that can be used to measure fixation disparity. How does their design differ?

2. List the major parameters of the FDC and, next to each parameter, give the findings that are likely to be associated with asthenopia.

3. Plot FDCs using the data on the next page. What are the curve type, slope, y-intercept, x-intercept, and center of symmetry for each curve?

Prism Setting (in Prism Diopters)	Fixation Disparity (in Minutes of Arc)			
	Patient JS	Patient CR	Patient JB	Patient RM
0	4 eso	2 eso	4 exo	0
3 base-in	8 eso	4 eso	2 exo	0
3 base-out	0	0	6 exo	0
6 base-in	14 eso	6 eso	0	4 eso
6 base-out	0	0	12 exo	2 exo
9 base-in	20 eso	10 eso	0	8 eso
9 base-out	4 exo	0	18 exo	4 exo
12 base-in	diplopia	20 eso	2 eso	12 eso
12 base-out	8 exo	0	25 exo	6 exo
15 base-in	diplopia	diplopia	2 eso	25 eso
15 base-out	20 exo	0	diplopia	12 exo
18 base-in	diplopia	diplopia	2 eso	diplopia
18 base-out	diplopia	0	diplopia	20 exo
21 base-in	diplopia	diplopia	diplopia	diplopia
21 base-out	diplopia	diplopia	diplopia	diplopia

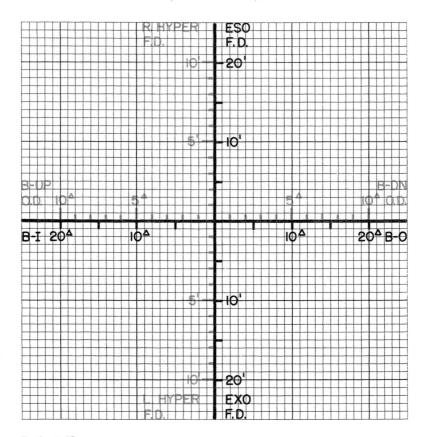

Patient JS

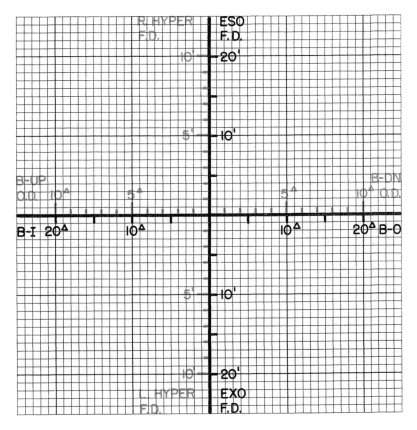

Patient CR

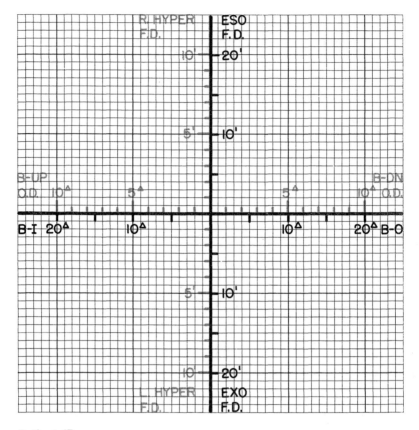

Patient JB

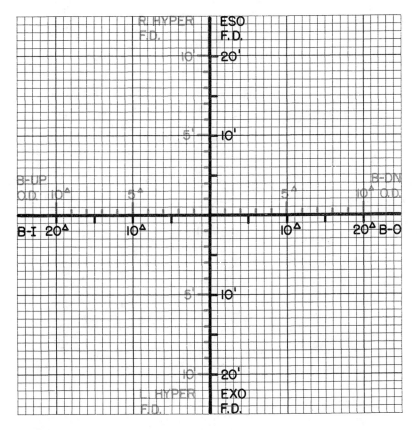

Patient RM

11

Prescription Guidelines for Vergence Disorder Case Types

A helpful first step in designing treatments for patients with convergence problems is to identify the vergence disorder case type. This is important because different diagnostic criteria are more effective in different case types[1-3] and because the efficacy of the different treatments for vergence disorders varies with the ACA ratio and direction of the phoria.[4,5] Lens adds are most effective when the ACA ratio is high. Among the various factors that increase the usefulness of prism prescriptions are moderate ACA ratio, so that the magnitude of the phorias is similar at distance and near, and, to a limited extent, esophoria as opposed to exophoria. Positive fusional vergence is easier to increase with vision training than is negative fusional vergence,[6,7] so vision training is more often the treatment of choice in exophoria than in esophoria.

The vergence disorder case types described below are (1) convergence insufficiency, (2) convergence excess, (3) divergence insufficiency, (4) divergence excess, (5) basic exo, (6) basic eso, (7) reduced fusional vergence, and (8) pseudoconvergence insufficiency. The ACA ratio is high in convergence excess and divergence excess, and low in convergence insufficiency and divergence insufficiency. Normal ACA ratios are found in basic exo, basic eso, and reduced fusional vergence case types. Pseudoconvergence insufficiency is an accommodative problem in which the patient exhibits dissociated phorias and some other findings similar to those in convergence insufficiency.

RECOMMENDED SYSTEM FOR ANALYSIS OF VERGENCE DISORDERS

We can use the above classification and the knowledge gained from the preceding chapters in a comprehensive approach to the analysis of vergence disorders. The steps in this system are as follows:

1. Use the normal ranges from Morgan's norms to determine whether the distance and near dissociated phorias are normal

(ortho to 2Δ exo at distance and ortho to 6Δ exo at near). Tentatively identify the case type based on the normalcy of the phorias.

2. Use the graph of the zone of clear single binocular vision (ZCSBV) to assess the pattern and consistency of findings. Use this information to confirm the case type classification.
3. Use the case type as a guide for the preferred method of treatment.
4. Use the analysis method appropriate to the case type as a guide in writing the prescription and designing the treatment program.

The following cases illustrate the application of this system in each of the case types.

Convergence Insufficiency

Convergence insufficiency is characterized by a normal distance phoria and a high exophoria at near. Other test results that help to identify cases of convergence insufficiency are low positive relative convergence (PRC) at near and a receded near point of convergence (NPC). The literature does not agree on a particular cut-off for the NPC to indicate convergence insufficiency,[8] but a general guideline is an NPC greater than 10 to 12 cm. The ACA ratio is low in convergence insufficiency. Accommodation findings are normal. Common symptoms of convergence insufficiency include ocular discomfort during reading and other near-point tasks, headaches, diplopia, blurred vision, and fatigue.[9,10] Some patients do not have asthenopia because they avoid near-point tasks.

The treatment of choice for convergence insufficiency is vision training to improve positive fusional vergence function. Vision training has a very high rate of success in relieving the symptoms of convergence insufficiency.[11–15] Grisham[15] summarized the results of several studies and reported that 72% of patients were "cured" and 91% of patients were either cured or improved with vision training. Successful vision training for convergence insufficiency is associated with an increase in PRC, a decrease in the NPC, and a flattening of the fixation disparity curve. A second, less desirable alternative is a prism prescription for near use.

An example of convergence insufficiency is given in Figure 11.1. We can use the steps above to analyze this case:

1. The distance phoria is within Morgan's norms. The near phoria is more exo than Morgan's norms. We can thus tentatively identify the case type as convergence insufficiency.
2. When we examine the graph of the ZCSBV (see Figure 11.1), we can see that the findings are consistent with each other in that

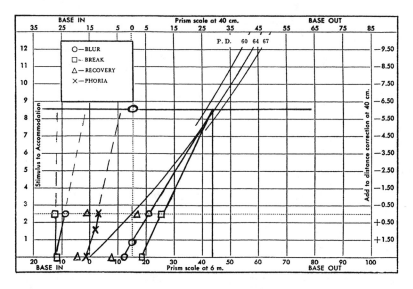

Figure 11.1 An example of convergence insufficiency. The complete graph is plotted from the following table.

	Phoria	Base-in	Base-out	Plus-to-Blur	Minus-to-Blur
6 m	1 exophoria	X/12/4	12/18/8		
40 cm	12 exophoria	24/28/16	6/10/2	+1.75	−6.00
40 cm + 1.00	13 exophoria				

Amplitude of accommodation = 8.50D; PD = 64 mm; NPC, = 12 cm.

the expected double parallelogram pattern of the ZCSBV is observed. We also can note that the PRC is low and the NPC is receded. The ACA ratio is low: calculated ACA = 1.6ΔD; gradient ACA = 1ΔD. Thus, we confirm convergence insufficiency.

3. The treatment of choice for convergence insufficiency is vision training.

4. In exophoria Sheard's criterion is useful and easily applied. The magnitude of the PRC should be twice the magnitude of the exophoria. In this case it is not, so the goal of the vision training program is to increase the base-out range to 24, which is twice the amount of the exophoria. If the patient is unwilling or unable to do vision training, a prism prescription based on the near associated phoria or the center of symmetry of the near fixation disparity curve can be used for reading and near-point activities.

Convergence Excess

Convergence excess is characterized by a normal distance phoria, esophoria at near, and a high calculated ACA ratio (greater than approximately 6Δ/D). A low negative relative convergence (NRC) finding is typical of convergence excess. Positive relative accommodation (PRA) often is low because of its relation to negative fusional vergence. Common symptoms of convergence excess include ocular discomfort and headaches following short periods of reading and occasional blurred vision or diplopia associated with near-point tasks. Convergence insufficiency and convergence excess are the most common vergence disorders.

The treatment of choice for convergence excess is to prescribe the subjective refraction for distance and a plus add for near.[16,17] A plus add is particularly effective because the ACA ratio is high. Another potential treatment is vision training to improve negative fusional vergence function. Although this is more difficult than improving positive fusional vergence, some clinicians have reported some success in increasing negative fusional vergence ranges.[7,18,19]

The amount of plus lens addition to prescribe can be derived using the near dissociated phoria and the gradient ACA ratio. The add should be the amount of plus that shifts the phoria to ortho or a small amount of exo (shifts it into the normal range). The plus add can be calculated using the following formula and then rounded up to the nearest 0.25D:

plus add = amount of esophoria/gradient ACA ratio

For example, if the near phoria is 7Δ eso and the gradient ACA ratio is 8Δ/D, the add would be +1.00D. Because the near phoria and the ACA ratio covary, the amount of the plus adds thus derived do not show much variation. Most adds for convergence excess are in the neighborhood of +1.00 or +1.25D.

Another way of deriving the power of the plus add is to use fixation disparity. The power of the add should be the minimum plus that reduces the eso fixation disparity to zero.

If vision training is undertaken, the 1:1 rule or Percival's criterion can be used to estimate the goal of the training program. Negative fusional vergence function should be improved to the extent to which these rules of thumb are met.

An example of convergence excess is shown in Figure 11.2. The distance phoria is normal and the near phoria is eso. These phorias, the high ACA ratio, and the pattern of the ZCSBV indicate convergence excess. The treatment of choice is a plus add. The near phoria through the subjective refraction to best visual acuity is 12Δ eso and the gradient ACA ratio is 11Δ/D, so the indicated add is +1.25D. If for some reason vision

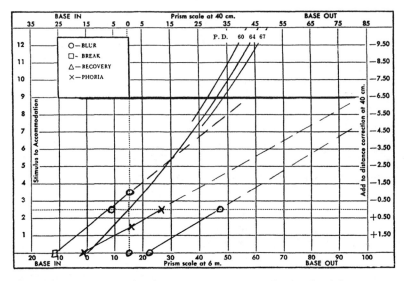

Figure 11.2 An example of convergence excess. The graph of the ZCSBV is plotted from the following table.

	Phoria	Base-in	Base-out	Plus-to-Blur	Minus-to-Blur
6 m	1 exophoria	X/12/6	22/28/16		
40 cm	12 esophoria	6/14/8	32/38/24	+2.50	−1.00
40 cm + 1.00	1 esophoria				

Amplitude of accommodation = 9.00D; PD = 66 mm.

training were to be undertaken in this case, the 1:1 rule would suggest that the base-in recovery at near should be increased to at least 12 (equal to the amount of the esophoria). Percival's criterion suggests that the goal of a vision training program would be to increase the base-in blur to at least 16 (half the amount of the base-out blur).

Divergence Insufficiency

Divergence insufficiency is characterized by esophoria at distance and a normal near phoria. The ACA ratio is low (calculated ACA ratio less than approximately 3Δ/D). Symptoms of divergence insufficiency include occasional diplopia at distance, headaches, and ocular discomfort.

The treatment of choice for divergence insufficiency is base-out prism.[16,20] Another alternative is vision training to improve negative fusional vergence. The base-out prism can be used only for distance or can be prescribed for full-time wear. Full-time wear is not a problem if the patient's positive fusional vergence capabilities are sufficient to handle the increased convergence stimulus at near; if not, it may be advisable to include vision training for both positive fusional vergence and negative fusional vergence along with the prism prescription. Prism can be prescribed from the distance-associated phoria.

Alteration of the spherical lens power is not a feasible approach in esophoria at distance, regardless of whether the ACA ratio is high or low, because accommodation should be at minimum levels while viewing at distance through the subjective refraction. Thus, an increase in plus power or a decrease in minus power over the subjective refraction will not decrease accommodation or accommodative convergence. However, when correcting the refractive error, it is advisable to prescribe the maximum plus to best visual acuity.

Figure 11.3 shows a case of divergence insufficiency. The distance phoria is a high eso and the near phoria is normal. The calculated ACA ratio is 1.6Δ/D and the gradient ACA ratio is 1Δ/D. The tilt of the ZCSBV is consistent with a low ACA ratio. In divergence insufficiency the treatment of choice is base-out prism. The distance-associated phoria indicates a prism prescription of 3Δ base-out. The 1:1 rule also would recommend a prism prescription of 3Δ base-out.

If the 3Δ base-out prism is worn full-time, it probably will not induce near problems. This prediction is based on the following reasoning. The near phoria through the subjective refraction is 2Δ exo. This represents a stimulus to positive fusional convergence of 2Δ. With the addition of a 3Δ base-out prism the stimulus to positive fusional convergence is 5. At near the positive fusional reserve convergence is 16 (the base-out blur at 40 cm through the subjective refraction). The 3Δ base-out prism will reduce the reserve by 3Δ to 13. With a demand of 5Δ and a reserve of 13Δ, Sheard's criterion would still be met. If vision training were to be undertaken, the goals would be to increase the base-in recovery at 6 m to at least 9Δ to satisfy the 1:1 rule and/or to increase the base-in break at 6 m to at least 13Δ to meet Percival's criterion.

Divergence Excess

Divergence excess is characterized by a high exophoria at distance and a normal-near phoria. The stimulus ACA ratio is high. Symptoms can include occasional diplopia at distance and asthenopia.[21]

Vision training for divergence excess is quite successful[12,21] and can be considered the treatment of choice. Base-in prism for distance and spherical lens adds also are potential options. Base-in prism can be prescribed using the distance-associated phoria. Since the ACA ratio is high,

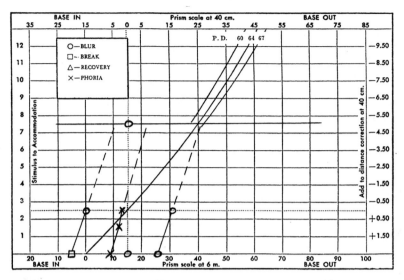

Figure 11.3 An example of divergence insufficiency. The graph of the ZCSBV is plotted from the following table.

	Phoria	Base-in	Base-out	Plus-to-Blur	Minus-to-Blur
6 m	9 esophoria	X/5/3	26/32/24		
40 cm	2 exophoria	15/20/12	16/24/12	+2.50	−5.00
40 cm + 1.00	3 exophoria				

Amplitude of accommodation = 7.50D; distance-associated phoria = 3Δ base-out; PD = 62 mm.

a decrease in plus power or an increase in minus power can be effective in reducing the distance exophoria. It should be kept in mind that the minus lens addition will make the near phoria as well the distance phoria more convergent. If the minus add induces an esophoria at near it may be advisable to prescribe a plus add at near in bifocal form.

Figure 11.4 illustrates a case of divergence excess. The distance phoria is high exo. The near phoria is within the normal range. The phoria line and the ZCSBV are tilted quite a bit to the right, indicating a high ACA ratio. The phorias and the pattern of the ZCSBV indicate divergence excess. The calculated ACA ratio is 8.8Δ/D. The gradient ACA ratio is 8Δ/D.

Sheard's criterion is met at 40 cm. Sheard's criterion is not met at 6 m. The treatment options available are base-out vision training, base-in prism at distance, and minus lens addition for distance. The goal of vi-

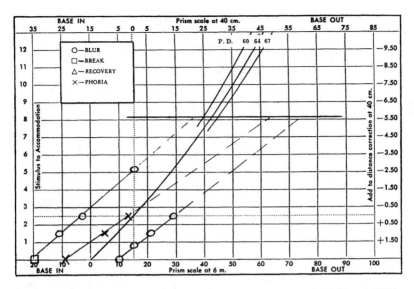

Figure 11.4 An example of divergence excess. The graph of the ZCSBV is plotted from the following table.

	Phoria	Base-in	Base-out	Plus-to-Blur	Minus-to-Blur
6 m	9 exophoria	X/20/12	10/16/6		
40 cm	2 exophoria	18/24/12	14/22/9	+1.75	−2.75
40 cm + 1.00	10 exophoria	26/30/18	6/14/2		

Amplitude of accommodation = 8.25D; distance-associated phoria = 3Δ base-in; PD = 64 mm.

sion training suggested by Sheard's criterion would be to increase the base-out limit to at least 18. Application of Sheard's criterion at 6 m suggests a prism prescription of approximately 2Δ base-in at distance. The distance-associated phoria gives the similar value of 3Δ base-in. Dividing 3Δ base-in by the gradient ACA ratio of 8Δ/D would indicate a lens addition of approximately −0.37D. Rounding to the next highest 0.25D would yield an add of −0.50D.

Basic Exophoria

Basic exophoria is characterized by greater than normal exophoria at both distance and near. The stimulus ACA ratio is at approximately normal levels. Base-out fusional vergence ranges may be lower than normal. The plus-to-blur finding may be low. Symptoms of basic exophoria may include eye strain or headaches associated with near work. The patient also may complain of occasional blurred vision or diplopia associated with either distance or near vision tasks.

Vision training for basic exophoria has a high rate of success[12,22] and is the treatment of choice for basic exophoria. If the associated phorias are similar in magnitude at distance and near, a base-in prism prescription from the associated phoria finding is a second alternative. The minus add from undercorrecting a hyperopia may be helpful if there is no accompanying accommodative problem.

A case of basic exophoria is shown in Figure 11.5. The distance and near dissociated phorias show a greater that normal amount of exopho-

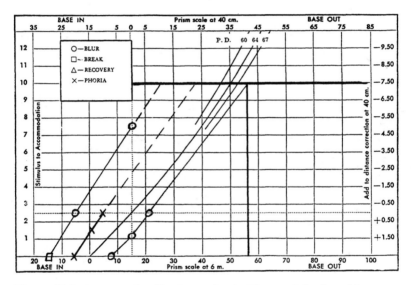

Figure 11.5 An example of basic exophoria. The graph is plotted from the following table.

	Phoria	Base-in	Base-out	Plus-to-Blur	Minus-to-Blur
6 m	7 exophoria	X/14/9	8/18/4		
40 cm	10 exophoria	20/28/14	6/20/2	+1.25	−5.00
40 cm + 1.00	14 exophoria				

Amplitude of accommodation = 10.00D; PD = 64 mm; NPC = 9 cm; distance-associated phoria = 3Δ base-in; near associated phoria = 4Δ base-in.

ria when compared with Morgan's normal ranges. The calculated ACA ratio is 4.8Δ/D. The gradient ACA ratio is 4Δ/D. The tilt of the ZCSBV looks normal, but it appears that the zone is shifted to the left. These findings indicate basic exophoria. Sheard's criterion is not met at either 6 m or 40 cm. The treatment of choice is vision training to increase positive fusional vergence. Improving the base-out limit so that Sheard's criterion is met would increase it to at least 14Δ at 6 m and at least 20Δ at 40 cm. The prism prescriptions suggested by Sheard's criterion are

6 m: P = 2/3(7) − 1/3(8) = 2Δ base-in

40 cm: P = 2/3(10) − 1/3(6) = 4 2/3Δ base-in

These are close to the associated phorias of 3Δ base-in at distance and 4Δ base-in at near. If the patient does not wish to do vision training a prism of approximately 3Δ base-in could be prescribed for full-time wear.

Basic Esophoria

In basic esophoria, esophoria is found at distance and near, and the ACA ratio is approximately normal. Base-in fusional vergence ranges may be lower than normal. The minus-to-blur finding may be low. Near-point asthenopia is a common complaint in basic esophoria. Symptoms also may include occasional blurred vision or diplopia during distance or near viewing.

The treatment of choice for basic esophoria is base-out prism. The prism can be prescribed using the associated phorias measured at distance and near. If the distance and near associated phorias are not equal, the lower amount of the two is usually prescribed. Another treatment option is vision training to improve negative fusional vergence. Hyperopic refractive error should be completely corrected.

If the amount of esophoria is significantly greater at near than at a distance, a plus add for near can be incorporated along with base-out prism or base-in vision training. This situation incorporates aspects of treatment of both basic esophoria and because the ACA ratio is high, convergence excess.

Figure 11.6 illustrates an example of basic esophoria. The dissociated phorias at distance and near show approximately equal amounts of esophoria. The base-in limits and the PRA are a little lower than normal. The calculated ACA ratio is 6.3Δ/D. The gradient ACA ratio is 6Δ/D. The tilt of the ZCSBV is approximately the same as the tilt of the demand line, but it appears shifted to the right compared with normal. These findings indicate basic esophoria.

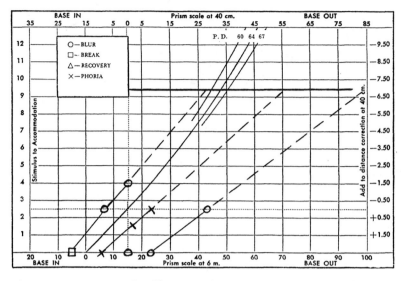

Figure 11.6 An example of basic esophoria. The graph is plotted from the following table.

	Phoria	Base-in	Base-out	Plus-to-Blur	Minus-to-Blur
6 m	7 esophoria	X/5/2	22/34/14		
40 cm	8 esophoria	8/14/4	28/38/17	+2.50	−1.50
40 cm + 1.00	2 esophoria				

Amplitude of accommodation = 9.50D; PD = 63 mm; distance-associated phoria = 3Δ base-out; near associated phoria = 3Δ base-out.

One way of managing basic esophoria is base-out prism. The prism recommended by Percival's criterion would be

6 m: P = 1/3(22) − 2/3(5) = 4Δ base-out
40 cm: P = 1/3(20) − 2/3(8) = 4Δ base-out

The prism recommended by the 1:1 rule would be

6 m: P = 7 − 2/2 = 2.5Δ base-out
40 cm: P = 8 − 4/2 = 2Δ base-out

These prism amounts are close to the associated phorias of 3Δ base-out at distance and 3Δ base-out at near. A prism of approximately 3Δ base-out can be prescribed.

Another mode of treatment in basic esophoria is vision training for negative fusional vergence. Percival's criterion suggests that the goal of vision training would be to increase the 6-m base-in limit to at least 11Δ and the 40-cm base-in limit to at least 14Δ. The 1:1 rule proposes that the goal of vision training would be to increase the base-in recoveries to at least 7Δ at 6 m and to at least 8Δ at 40 cm.

Reduced Fusional Vergence

In the reduced fusional vergence case type distance and near dissociated phorias are normal and the ACA ratio is normal, but both base-in and base-out fusional vergence ranges are below normal.[23,24] Amplitude of accommodation and lag of accommodation are normal. Asthenopic symptoms often are associated with reading or near work.

Treatment for reduced fusional vergence includes training to increase fusional vergence ranges in both directions to normal levels. The reduced fusional vergence function may be secondary to impediments to sensory fusion, such as uncorrected refractive error, aniseikonia, or suppression, or secondary to uncorrected vertical deviations.[25,26] Treatment should include correction of any accompanying refractive problems or vertical deviations.

The test findings in a case of reduced fusional vergence are shown in Figure 11.7. The dissociated phorias at both distance and near are normal. The calculated ACA ratio is 5.6Δ/D. The gradient ACA ratio is 4Δ/D. The tilt of the ZCSBV appears normal, but the zone is very narrow. The base-in limits, base-out limits, negative relative accommodation (NRA), and PRA are all low. The findings and the pattern of the ZCSBV indicate the reduced fusional vergence case type.

The treatment for reduced fusional vergence is vision training to improve both negative fusional vergence and positive fusional vergence. A reasonable goal is to increase the base-in and base-out limits to a point where they equal or exceed the mean values in Morgan's norms.

Pseudoconvergence Insufficiency

In pseudoconvergence insufficiency phoria findings are like those in convergence insufficiency: normal at distance and high exophoria at near. Positive relative convergence may be low or normal. Amplitude of accommodation is low. The lag of accommodation is abnormally high.

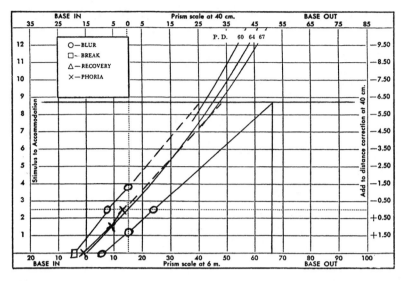

Figure 11.7 An example of reduced fusional vergence. The graph is plotted from the following table.

	Phoria	Base-in	Base-out	Plus-to-Blur	Minus-to-Blur
6 m	1 exophoria	X/4/2	6/12/4		
40 cm	2 exophoria	7/12/4	8/14/3	+1.25	−1.25
40 cm + 1.00	6 exophoria				

Amplitude of accommodation = 8.75; PD = 64 mm; near-point of convergence = 7 cm.

Examination of the ZCSBV shows that the left and right sides of the zone show a normal amount of tilt to the right. The phoria line is less tilted than the sides of the zone.[17] As discussed in Chapter 4, this occurs because accommodation is reduced, and thus accommodative vergence is reduced during measurement of the near phoria. The ACA ratio appears low because the lag of accommodation is abnormally high when the near phoria is taken. The NPC is receded. An interesting phenomenon that occurs in pseudoconvergence insufficiency is that the NPC improves with a plus add.[27] This paradoxical result is thought to be due to increased accommodative accuracy with the plus add, allowing accommodation and accommodative convergence to increase as the target is moved closer to the patient. Pseudoconvergence insufficiency actually is an accommodative insufficiency rather than a "true" convergence insufficiency. Therefore, treatment is aimed at managing the accommodative problem. A high lag of accommodation usually is treated with a plus add for near-point. A secondary treatment is vision training to improve accommodative function. If the vision training is successful the phoria will tilt over further to the right so that it roughly parallels the left and right sides of the ZCSBV. An example of pseudoconvergence insufficiency was shown previously in Figure 4.1.

COMMENTS AND OTHER CONSIDERATIONS

The guidelines above are for patients without strabismus or sensory anomalies such as amblyopia. Most of the same basic principles apply to patients with strabismus, but treatment also must include training for sensory anomalies, such as amblyopia, suppression, etc.[28-30]

There have been many different schemes proposed by various investigators for establishing the phoria levels that define each of the vergence disorder case types. The classification scheme described above is probably the easiest to remember because it is based on the well-known Morgan normal ranges for phorias. The identification of a treatment of choice for each of the case types is based on the principles that phorias are most easily shifted to normal levels by lens adds when the ACA ratio is high and that vision training usually is more effective in improving positive fusional vergence than negative fusional vergence. The phorias, ZCSBV pattern, recommended treatment, and preferred analysis methods for each of the vergence disorder types are summarized in Table 11.1.

The efficacy of prism correction in relieving oculomotor symptoms has received only limited controlled study. In a study by Worrell et al,[31] subjects wore either glasses without prism or identical-appearing glasses with prism, as indicated by Sheard's criterion. The subjects participated in the study for 2 weeks, wearing one type of glasses the first week and the other type the following week. At the end of this time the subjects indicated which glasses they preferred. Although the sample size was small, the results suggested that prism corrections are best tolerated in esophoria at distance. The results also suggested that presbyopes with exo deviations at near tolerate prisms, but younger persons do not. Payne et al[32] described a study in which 10 symptomatic patients preferred spectacles prescribed from near Mallet unit-associated phorias over spectacles with no prism. Each pair of spectacles was worn for 1 week. Nine of the 10 subjects had exo fixation disparity at near. Carter[33] noted that when prism is given to a person who exhibits prism adaptation, that individual indicates a need for a larger prism at the next examination. He proposes that this should not be a problem if the optometrist does not prescribe prism for an asymptomatic person or for

Table 11.1

Summary of signs, preferred analysis method, and recommended treatment for each of the vergence disorder case types.

Case Type	Distance Phoria	Near Phoria	ACA Ratio	Other Important Findings	Pattern of ZCSBV	Treatment of Choice	Analysis Method Outcome Correlated With Symptoms	Prescription or Vision Training Goal
Convergence Insufficiency	normal	high exo	low	receded NPC, normal accommodation, (low N' PRC')	less tilted to right than normal	base-out vision training	Sheard's criterion not met at near	VT: increase near PRC to at least twice the near exophoria
Convergence Excess	normal	eso	high	low NRC at near, low PRA	more tilted to right than normal	plus add at near	greater esophoria, 1:1 rule not met at near, Percival's criterion not met at near	plus add which makes near phoria ortho or low exo; or plus add which reduces fixation disparity to zero
Divergence Insufficiency	eso	normal	low	low NRC at distance	distance portion shifted to right compared with normal, less tilted than normal	base-out prism for distance or vision training	greater esophoria, 1:1 rule not met at distance, Percival's criterion not met at distance	prism: distance associated phoria; VT: increase NRC at distance so that 1:1 rule met, Percival's criterion met
Divergence Excess	high exo	normal	high	low PRC at distance	distance portion shifted to left compared with normal; more tilted than normal	base-out vision training	Sheard's criterion not met at distance	VT: increase distance PRC to at least twice the near exophoria: or minus add to make distance phoria normal
Basic Exophoria	high exo	high exo	moderate	low PRC at distance and near, low NRA	entire zone shifted to left compared with normal	base-out vision training	Sheard's criterion not met at distance and/or near	VT: increase distance and near PRC values to at least twice the respective amounts of exophoria
Basic Esophoria	eso	eso	moderate	low NRC at distance and near, low PRA	entire zone shifted to right compared with normal	base-out prism	greater esophoria, 1:1 rule and/or Percival's criterion not met at distance and/or near	prism prescription from distance and near associated phorias
Reduced Fusional Vergence	normal	normal	normal	fusional vergence ranges low: vergence facility low; NRA and PRA low	positive and negative widths both less than normal; tilt normal	vision training	NRC and PRC lower than normal	VT: increase NRC and PRC to normal levels
Pseudo Convergence Insufficiency	normal	high exo	appears low due to poor accommodation response	reduced NPC; NPC improves with plus add; amplitude of accommodation low; lag of accommodation high	tilt of left and right sides normal; phoria line less tilted than normal	plus add	abnormal accommodation findings	plus add according to accommodation findings

an individual without a significant distance heterophoria. Prism adaptation also can be tested for by remeasuring the phorias after the patient reads for a few minutes while using the proposed prism prescription. A significant change in the phorias indicates prism adaptation, in which case the prescription may be contraindicated. It has been proposed that the use of fixation disparity and associated phorias for prescribing prism is effective because fixation disparity is affected by prism adaptation.[34]

The most common method for measuring phorias is the von Graefe prism dissociation technique. If there is some question about the validity of a phoria measurement using the von Graefe technique with the refractor, then the measurement should be repeated and/or other subjective and objective testing methods (such as stereoscope, Maddox rod, and cover test prism neutralization) should be used. It also should be verified that in high refractive errors an inaccurate phoria measurement is not the result of a tilt of the refractor or the use of an improper interpupillary distance.

As mentioned, if the ACA ratio is high, spherical lens power alterations will be effective in changing convergence posture. Since this is not true for patients with low ACA ratios, prism correction or vision training is preferable to lens power changes when the ACA ratio is low. Prism correction is more practically incorporated in spectacles for full-time wear if the ACA ratio is moderate and thus the phorias are similar at different distances. Spherical lens power alterations that would compromise clear vision or a comfortable range of accommodation should not be used.

When using a device that measures only associated phorias (as opposed to the entire fixation disparity curve), a prism prescription can be based on the associated phoria. However, Disparometer fixation disparity curve x-intercepts are greater in magnitude than Bernell unit and Borish card near-associated phorias.[35] Using the entire fixation disparity curve, the prism prescription should be based on the center of symmetry. Prescriptions are made primarily when the patient is experiencing asthenopia or withdraws from visual tasks. Obviously, a careful case history[36-38] is indispensable in evaluating the patient's visual needs and complaints.

Case Report: Patient AG

AG, an 11-year-old boy, complained of blurred near vision. He stated that letters ran together. He did not wear spectacles. Unaided visual acuities were 6/6–2/6 OD, 6/6 OS, 6/6–2/6 OU at distance, and 20/20–2/8 OD, 20/20–3/8 OS at near. The cover test showed orthophoria at distance and a small esophoria at near. Near point of convergence was to the nose. The subjective refraction was plano D sphere OU. Salient examination findings are shown in Figure 11.8. The phoria find-

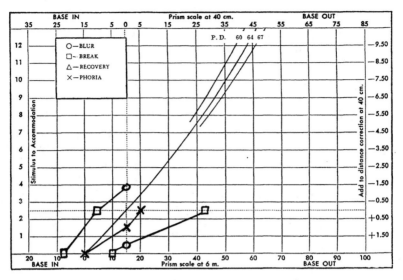

Figure 11.8 The following test results were obtained for patient AG.

	Phoria	Base-in	Base-out	Plus-to-Blur	Minus-to-Blur
6 m	orthophoria	X/8/4	X/10/0		
40 cm	5 esophoria	X/10/2	X/28/20	+2.00	−1.25
40 cm + 1.00	orthophoria				

PD = 59 mm; eso fixation disparity at 40 cm with plano sphere OU, zero fixation disparity with +1.00D sphere OU.

ings and the high ACA ratio suggest convergence excess. This is confirmed by noting the low base-in findings at near, the low PRA, and the fact that the ZCSBV tilts to the right, as shown in Figure 11.8. It may be noted that the 1:1 rule is not met at 40 cm. A +1.00D add was sufficient to shift the esophoria at near to orthophoria. An eso fixation disparity was noted with no lenses in place. Fixation disparity was reduced to zero with +1.00D spheres. The patient was asked to look at magazine print with +1.00D lenses held in front of his eyes, and he stated that he could read finer print with the lenses. It also was demonstrated that these lenses made distance vision blurry. The options of single vision reading lenses, bifocals, and progressive addition lenses were explained to AG and his family, and they decided on single vision reading lenses. Lenses with powers of +1.00D sphere were prescribed. AG subsequently reported that he could read much more easily with his spectacles.

Case Report: Patient FN

Patient FN, a 28-year-old female graduate student, complained of afternoon headaches, a vague tiredness around the eyes, and a pulling sensation around the eyes. She had 1-year-old glasses for distance vision which she wore on a full-time basis. The glasses were −2.25–0.50 × 175 OD, −2.25–0.25 × 10 OS. Distance visual acuities with these lenses were 6/4.5–2/6 OD, 6/4.5–3/6 OS, 6/4.5–1/6 OU. Aided near acuities were 20/20 OD and OS. The cover test with the habitual correction revealed orthophoria at distance and a moderately large exophoria at near.

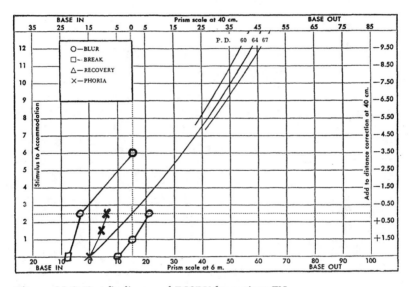

Figure 11.9 Test findings and ZCSBV for patient FN.

	Phoria	Base-in	Base-out	Plus-to-Blur	Minus-to-Blur
6 m	orthophoria	X/8/4	10/18/6		
40 cm	9 exophoria	18/22/12	6/18/0	+1.50	−3.50
40 cm + 1.00	11 exophoria				

PD = 62 mm; amplitude of accommodation = 10.00D.

The NPC was 9 cm. The subjective refraction was $-2.50-0.25 \times 170$ OD (6/4.5–1/6), $-2.25-0.25 \times 15$ OS (6/4.5–1/6). This patient's ZCSBV is shown in Figure 11.9. The phorias, the receded NPC, the low PRC, the low NRA, and the pattern of the ZCSBV indicate convergence insufficiency. It may be noted that Sheard's criterion was not met at 40 cm. The patient was started on a vision training program that included daily at-home work on a Brock string and Tranaglyphs and once-a-week office visits for additional training. After 4 weeks, the patient reported that her headaches and eyestrain were much less frequent. The base-out fusional vergence range at 40 cm had improved to 20/27/8, the NRA had improved to +2.00D, and the NPC was found to be 4.5 cm.

REFERENCES

1. Sheedy JE, Saladin JJ. Phoria, vergence, and fixation disparity in oculomotor problems. *Am J Optom Physiol Opt.* 1977;54:474–478.
2. Sheedy JE, Saladin JJ. Association of symptoms with measures of oculomotor deficiencies. *Am J Optom Physiol Opt.* 1978;55:670– 676.
3. Sheedy JE, Saladin JJ. Validity of diagnostic criteria and case analysis in binocular vision disorders. In: Schor C M, Ciuffreda K J, eds. *Vergence Eye Movements: Basic and Clinical Aspects.* Boston, MA: Butterworth-Heinemann; 1983:517–540.
4. Scheiman M, Wick B. *Clinical Management of Binocular Vision—Heterophoric, Accommodative, and Eye Movement Disorders.* Philadelphia, PA: Lippincott; 1994: 87–100.
5. Saladin JJ. Horizontal prism prescription. In: Cotter SA, ed. *Clinical Uses of Prism–A Spectrum of Applications—Mosby's Optometric Problem Solving Series.* St Louis, MO: Mosby-Year Book. 1995:109–147.
6. Morgan MW. Analysis of clinical data. *Am J Optom Arch Am Acad Optom.* 1944;21:477–491.
7. Daum KM. The course and effect of visual training on the vergence system. *Am J Optom Physiol Opt.* 1982;59:223–227.
8. Daum KM. Characteristics of convergence insufficiency. *Am J Optom Physiol Opt.* 1988;65:426–438.
9. Cooper J, Duckman R. Convergence insufficiency: incidence, diagnosis, and treatment. *J Am Optom Assoc.* 1978;49:673–680.
10. Daum KM. Convergence insufficiency. *Am J Optom Physiol Opt.* 1984;61:16–22.
11. Cooper J, Selenow A, Ciuffreda KJ, et al. Reduction of asthenopia in patients with convergence insufficiency after fusional vergence training. *Am J Optom Physiol Opt.* 1983;60:982–989.
12. Daum KM. Characteristics of exodeviations. II. Changes with treatment with orthoptics. *Am J Optom Physiol Opt.* 1986;63:244–251.
13. Suchoff IB, Petito GT. The efficacy of visual therapy: accommodative disorders and non-strabismic anomalies of binocular vision. *J Am Optom Assoc.* 1986;57:119–125.
14. Griffin JR. Efficacy of vision therapy for nonstrabismic vergence anomalies. *Am J Optom Physical Opt.* 1987;64:411–414.

15. Grisham JD. Visual therapy results for convergence insufficiency: a literature review. *Am J Optom Physiol Opt.* 1988;65:448–454.
16. Wick BC. Horizontal deviations. In: Amos JF, ed. *Diagnosis and Management in Vision Care.* Boston, MA: Butterworth-Heinemann; 1987:461–510.
17. Grosvenor TP. *Primary Care Optometry.* 2nd ed. New York, NY: Professional Press; 1989:343–346.
18. Daum KM. Negative vergence training in humans. *Am J Optom Physiol Opt.* 1986;63:487–496.
19. Shorter AD, Hatch SW. Vision therapy for convergence excess. *N Engl J Optom.* 1993;45:51–53.
20. Scheiman M, Gallaway M, Ciner E. Divergence insufficiency: characteristics, diagnosis, and treatment. *Am J Optom Physiol Opt.* 1986;63:425–431.
21. Daum KM. Divergence excess: characteristics and results of treatment with orthoptics. *Ophthal Physiol Opt.* 1984;4:15–24.
22. Daum KM. Equal exodeviations: characteristics and results of treatment with orthoptics. *Aust J Optom.* 1984;67:53–59.
23. Grisham JD. The dynamics of fusional vergence eye movements in binocular dysfunction. *Am J Optom Physiol Opt.* 1980;57:645–655.
24. Grisham JD. Treatment of binocular dysfunctions. In: Schor CM, Ciuffreda KJ, eds. *Vergence Eye Movements: Basic and Clinical Aspects.* Boston, MA: Butterworth-Heinemann; 1983:605–646.
25. Schapero M. The characteristics of ten basic visual training problems. *Am J Optom Arch Am Acad Optom.* 1955;32:333–342.
26. Scheiman M, Wick B. *Clinical Management of Binocular Vision—Heterophoric, Accommodative, and Eye Movement Disorders.* Philadelphia, PA: Lippincott; 1994:308–311.
27. Richman JE, Cron MT. *Guide to Vision Therapy.* South Bend, IN: Bernell Corporation; 1987:17–18.
28. Griffin JR. *Binocular Anomalies—Procedures for Vision Therapy.* 2nd ed. Boston, MA: Butterworth-Heinemann; 1982.
29. von Noorden GK. *Binocular Vision and Ocular Motility—Theory and Management of Strabismus.* 4th ed. St Louis, MO: Mosby; 1990.
30. Caloroso EE, Rouse MW. *Clinical Management of Strabismus.* Boston, MA: Butterworth-Heinemann; 1993.
31. Worrell BE Jr, Hirsch MJ, Morgan MW. An evaluation of prism prescribed by Sheard's criterion. *Am J Optom Arch Am Acad Optom.* 1971;48:373–376.
32. Payne CR, Grisham JD, Thomas KL. A clinical evaluation of fixation disparity. *Am J Optom Physiol Opt.* 1974;51:88–90.
33. Carter DB. Effects of prolonged wearing of prism. *Am J Optom Arch Am Acad Optom.* 1963;40:265–273.
34. Schor CM. Fixation disparity and vergence adaptation. In: Schor CM, Ciuffreda KJ, eds. *Vergence Eye Movements: Basic and Clinical Aspects.* Boston, MA: Butterworth-Heinemann; 1983:465–516.
35. Brownlee GA, Goss DA. Comparisons of commercially available devices for the measurement of fixation disparity and associated phorias. *J Am Optom Assoc.* 1988;59:451–460.
36. Borish IM. *Clinical Refraction.* 3rd ed. Chicago, IL: Professional Press; 1970:307–344.
37. Grosvenor TP. *Primary Care Optometry.* 2nd ed. Boston, MA: Butterworth-Heinemann; 1989:119–136.

38. Birnbaum MH. *Optometric Management of Nearpoint Vision Disorders*. Boston, MA: Butterworth-Heinemann; 1993:89–96.

SUGGESTED READING

Grisham JD. Treatment of binocular dysfunctions. In: Schor CM, Ciuffreda KJ, eds. *Vergence Eye Movements: Basic and Clinical Aspects*. Boston, MA: Butterworth-Heinemann; 1983:605–646.
Grosvenor T. Binocular vision syndromes. *Optom Weekly*. 1975;66:803–808.
Grosvenor T. The use of the AC/A ratio in prescribing. *Optom Weekly*. 1975;66:726–728.
Saladin JJ. Horizontal prism prescription. In: Cotter SA, ed. *Clinical Uses of Prism—A Spectrum of Applications Mosby's Optometric Problem Solving Series*. St Louis, MO: Mosby-Year Book. 1995:109–147.
Schapero M. The characteristics of ten basic visual training problems. *Am J Optom Arch Acad Optom*. 1955;32:333–342.

PRACTICE PROBLEMS

Plot all the findings for the following patients. Identify any erroneous findings, calculate the ACA ratios, and do the necessary calculations for Sheard's and Percival's criteria. Are the findings characteristic of any of the binocular vision syndromes? Indicate what you would prescribe and why. Unless otherwise noted, all findings are through the distance subjective refraction.

	Patient PR 64-mm PD	Patient ST 64-mm PD	Patient RK 60-mm PD	Patient EN 62-mm PD	Patient CD 65-mmPD
Amplitude of accommodation	5.00D	6.50D	12.00D	9.00D	7.50D
6 m phoria	orthophoria	orthophoria		8 esophoria	
6 m base-in	X/10/4	X/8/4		X/6/0	
6 m base-out	12/16/8	26/30/20		20/28/8	
4 m phoria			8 exophoria		12 exophoria
4 m base-in			X/18/12		X/20/14
4 m base-out			8/24/12		X/10/6
40 cm phoria	9 exophoria	12 esophoria	12 exophoria	4 exophoria	2 exophoria
40 cm base-in	22/26/18	7/12/2	26/30/14	14/18/4	16/28/12

	Patient PR 64-mm PD	Patient ST 64-mm PD	Patient RK 60-mm PD	Patient EN 62-mm PD	Patient CD 65-mmPD
40 cm base-out	6/12/3	32/38/20	10/30/16	16/30/12	25/36/16
40 cm plus-to-blur	+2.00	+2.50	+1.50	+2.50	+2.00
40 cm minus-to-blur	−2.50	−1.25	−5.50	−5.25	−2.00
40 cm + 1.00 add phoria	11 exophoria	2 esophoria	16 exophoria	5 exophoria	12 exophoria
40 cm + 1.00 add base-in	X/24/16	16/24/11	X/30/20	16/20/16	26/32/20
40 cm + 1.00 add base-out	2/10/0	24/32/14	6/24/18	12/24/8	16/34/8
40 cm − 1.00 add phoria			7 exophoria	orthophoria	5 esophoria
40 cm − 1.00 add base-in			24/28/16	14/20/12	
40 cm − 1.00 add base-out			6/32/20	24/34/16	

For the test findings in the following table:

1. Graph the findings.
2. What is the calculated ACA ratio?
3. What is the gradient ACA ratio?
4. What are the amounts of NRC, negative fusional convergence, PRC, and positive fusional convergence at 40 cm?
5. What is the demand on fusional convergence and the reserve at 6 cm?
6. What is the demand on fusional convergence and the reserve at 40 cm?
7. What is the positive width of the ZCSBV at 40 cm?
8. What is the negative width of the ZCSBV at 40 cm?
9. Is Sheard's criterion met at 6 m? Is it met at 40 cm? If not, what prism, lens add, or vision training end point would be necessary to meet it?
10. Is Percival's criterion met at 6 m? Is it met at 40 cm? If not, what prism, lens add, or vision training end point would be necessary to meet it?

11. Is the 1:1 rule met at 6 m? Is it met at 40 cm? If not, what prism, lens add, or vision training end point would be necessary to meet it?
12. Which of the vergence disorder case types do the findings indicate?
13. What is the treatment of choice for this case type?
14. Why is that the treatment of choice for this case type?

All test findings were taken through the distance subjective refraction except for near phorias taken through a +1.00D add as noted.

	Patient TS 64-mm PD	Patient DN 63-mm PD	Patient DH 62-mm PD	Patient BP 64-mm PD	Patient ST 66-mm PD
Amplitude of accommodation	15.00D	11.00D	8.25D	11.50D	8.75D
Convergence amplitude	90Δ	>100Δ	46Δ	92Δ	51Δ
6 m phoria	ortho	2 exo	4 exo	3 eso	1 exo
6 m base-in	X/8/4	X/12/6	X/8/6	X/7/2	X/7/3
6 m base-out	24/40/14	18/22/10	8/10/6	18/24/4	8/20/6
40 cm phoria	12 eso	4 eso	8 eso	3 eso	9 exo
40 cm + 1.00 phoria	3 eso	8 exo	12 exo	2 eso	11 eso
40 cm base-in	8/18/4	18/24/14	12/24/18	12/18/2	18/22/15
40 cm base-out	32/40/24	20/24/18	4/12/−2	20/27/8	12/27/8
40 cm plus-to-blur	+2.50	+2.50	+1.00	+2.50	+1.50
40 cm minus-to-blur	−1.25	−3.25	−3.75	−1.75	−6.25

	Patient JJ 64-mm PD	Patient GB 60-mm PD	Patient MS 64-mm PD	Patient RS 63-mm PD
Amplitude of accommodation	7.50D	11.75D	10.00D	9.50D
Convergence amplitude	81Δ	100Δ	83Δ	70Δ
6 m phoria	4 eso	1 exo	6 exo	ortho
6 m base-in	X/6/0	X/10/4	X/14/8	X/3/2
6 m base-out	22/28/18	12/28/6	6/18/2	7/14/6
40 cm phoria	2 exo	4 exo	1 exo	1 exo
40 cm + 1.00 phoria	5 exo	8 exo	8 exo	4 exo
40 cm base-in	14/18/10	14/20/7	15/22/8	6/10/2
40 cm base-out	18/25/12	20/33/12	24/34/10	8/15/4
40 cm plus-to-blur	+2.50	+2.25	+1.75	+1.50
40 cm minus-to-blur	−5.00	−3.75	−2.00	−1.00

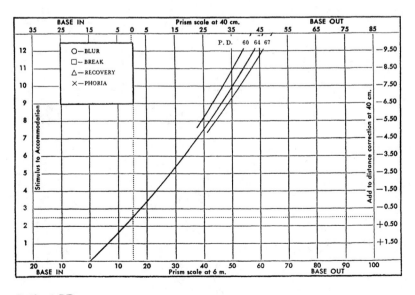

Patient PR

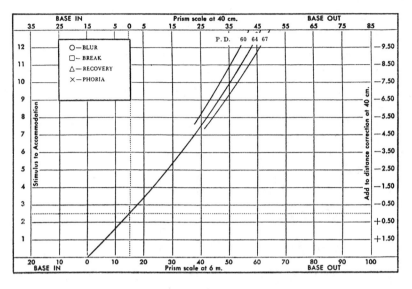

Patient ST

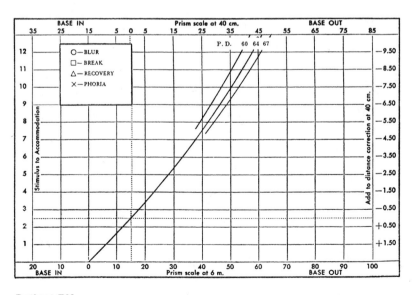

Patient RK

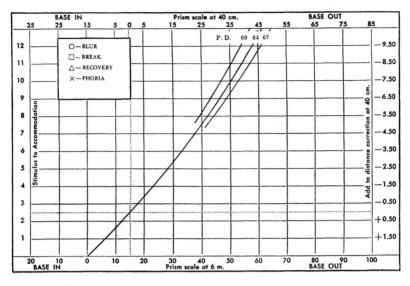

Patient EN

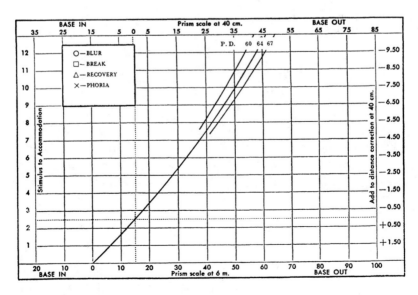

Patient CD

12

Presbyopia

Presbyopia is "a reduction in accommodative ability occurring normally with age and necessitating a plus lens addition for satisfactory seeing at near, sometimes quantitatively identified by the recession of the near-point of accommodation beyond 20 cm."[1] The primary symptom of presbyopia is blurred near vision or difficulty reading fine print. Patients often report that they get some improvement in clarity of reading material by holding it further away. Patients occasionally state that their eyes "pull" or feel strained when trying to read. The defining sign of presbyopia is reduced amplitude of accommodation.

AMPLITUDE OF ACCOMMODATION

Amplitude of accommodation is "the difference expressed in diopters between the far point and the near-point of accommodation with respect to the spectacle plane, the entrance pupil, or some other reference point of the eye."[2] Generally, the amplitude of accommodation is measured by noting the distance from the punctum proximum or near-point of accommodation to the spectacle plane while the patient wears the correction for ametropia. The near-point of accommodation usually is determined by a push-up test performed monocularly with each eye and binocularly, and it is the closest of the three measurements thus derived.[3,4] The distance measured can then be converted into diopters. If the patient is not wearing lenses equal to the subjective refraction during the test, then adjustment must be made to the dioptric value obtained: an increase if insufficient plus is worn, a decrease if insufficient minus is worn. A formula for amplitude of accommodation in diopters is as follows:

$$\text{Amplitude of accommodation} = \frac{100}{\text{NPA in cm}} + [\text{RE} - \text{L}]$$

where NPA represents the near-point of accommodation (usually measured in cm), RE represents the patient's refractive error in diopters, and L represents the power in diopters of the lens worn while the measurement of the near-point of accommodation was taken.

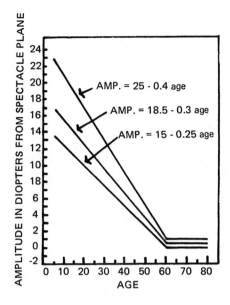

Figure 12.1
The relationship between amplitude
of accommodation in diopters and age
in years, according to Hofstetter's
formulas.
(Reprinted with permission from H.W.
Hofstetter. A useful age-amplitude
formula. *Pennsylvania Optom.* 1947;7:5–8.)

There is a predictable gradual decline in amplitude throughout one's life. Various tables of amplitude norms for given ages are available. Formulas for the expected changes in amplitude of accommodation with age also can be used. Hofstetter[5,6] derived the following formulas (also shown in Figure 12.1) for amplitude from the data of Donders, Duane, and Kaufman:

Maximum amplitude $= 25 - 0.4$ age
Probable amplitude $= 18.5 - 0.3$ age
Minimum amplitude $= 15 - 0.25$ age

These formulas are applicable up to 60 years of age. At approximately 60 years of age, absolute presbyopia, the condition in which accommodative ability is completely absent,[1] has been reached. The normal range of amplitudes of accommodation for persons 60 years of age and over is 0 to 1.00D.[6] Patients with absolute presbyopia often will have amplitude of accommodation measurements up to 1.00D because of the depth of focus of the eye.

RULES AND TESTS FOR PRESCRIBING PRESBYOPIC ADDS

Various rules of thumb can be applied, along with a consideration of the patient's needs and preferences and the previous prescription, to determine the power of the add to be prescribed.[7-11] One such rule is to keep half the amplitude in reserve. In other words, for most visual tasks the patient should not be required to use more than half the amplitude of accommodation. The use of this rule necessitates the accurate determination of the patient's habitual preferred working distances. A formula for the rule can be written as follows:

Add = Stimulus to accommodation at working distance
$\qquad$ − amplitude of accommodation/2

For instance, if an individual's usual working distance is 40 cm and the amplitude of accommodation is 1.50D, the add proposed by this rule is calculated as

$$\text{Add} = \frac{100}{40 \text{ cm}} - \frac{1.50D}{2}$$
$$= 2.50D - 0.75D$$
$$= 1.75D$$

A second rule used to determine an add involves balancing the plus-lens-to-blur (negative relative accommodation [NRA]) and the minus-lens-to-blur (positive relative accommodation [PRA]) findings. It states that the proper add allows the plus-lens-to-blur value to be equal to the minus-lens-to-blur value; if this value cannot be achieved by an add that is a multiple of 0.25D, then the plus-lens-to-blur should be 0.25D larger than the minus-lens-to-blur. The qualifier at the end of the statement is used because adds are available only in 0.25D steps. It is implied that this criterion refers to the patient's usual working distance. As long as the minus-to-blur and plus-to-blur points on the graph fall at the top (amplitude of accommodation line) and bottom of the zone of clear single binocular vision (ZCSBV), respectively, rather than at the left and right sides of the ZCSBV, respectively, the add proposed by this rule will be the same as the add proposed by keeping half the amplitude in reserve. An example of the use of the rule is

Working distance = 40 cm
Plus-lens-to-blur taken at 40 cm through +2.00 add = +0.50D
Minus-lens-to-blur taken at 40 cm through +2.00 add = −1.00D
Add suggested = +1.75D

If a +1.75D add is used, the result will be an interval of 0.75D to both the plus-to-blur and minus-to-blur.

The near binocular cross cylinder (BCC) test yields the lens power with which the retina is conjugate to the test target. Some practitioners use the BCC test to derive a tentative presbyopic add, which then can be refined by additional testing, such as the NRA, PRA, and accommodative ranges. By itself, the BCC often will give an add power that is too high for a beginning presbyope, but is quite close to the final prescription for the advanced presbyope.

Another useful test is the plus build-up test. The test is started with the distance subjective refraction lenses. The patient is instructed to look at the 20/20 letters or letters at the patient's best acuity level on a reduced Snellen card at 40 cm or the patient's usual working distance. Plus is added in 0.25D steps. The patient is instructed to report when the letters are first readable. The clinician notes this add amount. Then more plus is added in 0.25D steps, and the patient reports when the letters are seen most clearly. This lens power can be refined by additional add testing, such as the NRA, PRA, and accommodative ranges. The final prescription is usually 0.50D more plus than the "first readable" lens add level on the plus build-up test. The final prescription usually is equal to the patient's preferred add level on the plus build-up test.

There are other less popular rules of thumb that can be used to suggest an add, and there are many intangible factors to consider. As a result, it is difficult to identify a single rule of thumb as being used consistently by most optometrists.[12] Such subjective factors as the patient's previous prescription, visual symptoms, and habitual working distance must be taken into account.[8,11] Patients' complaints that they must hold near-work farther away than they would like indicate that an increase in plus power is advisable, whereas large lens power changes when patients are satisfied with a previous prescription may cause patient dissatisfaction, regardless of the fact that the change may be indicated by a rule of thumb. Morgan[13] and Patorgis[8] have given detailed discussions of these factors.

ACCOMMODATIVE RANGES

An additional test that some practitioners use is the measurement of accommodative ranges through the near correction.[14] This test involves the determination of a near-point and far-point of accommodation through the proposed near correction. The patient's working distance should be closer to the patient than the middle of the near range for the results to correlate with the rules of thumb discussed earlier.

Since a range of accommodation (linear distance from near-point to far-point) is not directly converted into amplitude of accommodation in diopters, the data obtained from the ranges cannot be directly interpreted to yield a value for an add. All that can be said is that the patient's working distance should be nearer than the midpoint of the range. The actual purpose of the test, as used by most practitioners, is as a demonstration to the patient that the results of previous testing are confirmed.[14] Most commonly, the tentative near-point prescription is placed in a trial frame, and subjective comments as well as the near-point and far-point are elicited by moving the test card farther away and nearer. The add is then increased or decreased to alter the range.

RELATIONSHIP OF PRESCRIBED ADD TO AGE

Since the amplitude of accommodation declines with age, the power of the presbyopic reading addition will increase with age. Several texts contain tables with expected add as a function of age.[7,8,11] It is helpful to consider age as a factor to check the proposed add, but the clinician should not rely on age over carefully performed testing in prescribing adds for presbyopia.[7,11]

ZONE OF CLEAR SINGLE BINOCULAR VISION IN PRESBYOPIA

The presbyopic ZCSBV may show only a decrease in height without any other apparent change in the five fundamental variables of the zone.[15] Associated either directly or indirectly with the decrease in amplitude of accommodation are several apparent variations in the results of conventional clinic tests:

1. An increase in exophoria or a decrease in esophoria in the near-point tests attributable to a lower amount of accommodative convergence, since a plus add substitutes for accommodation.

2. An increase in the near-point base-in blur, break, and recovery and a decrease in the base-out blur, break, and recovery also resulting from the reduction in accommodative convergence associated with the plus add.

3. The base-out limit possibly showing a break without a blur because the presbyope may not be able to accommodate sufficiently to obtain a blur on this test.

4. A lower minus-lens-to-blur directly attributable to the reduction in the amplitude of accommodation.

5. The possible addition of a rightward extension to the upper right corner of the zone. This tail, or spike, occurs only in some individuals, and only when a base-out limit is taken at a stimulus

to accommodation level at or near the patient's amplitude of accommodation. One possible explanation for the tail is that a greater accommodative convergence occurs because an increased innervation to accommodation is necessary for an accommodative response at or near the amplitude.[16,17]

Since the height of the ZCSBV is reduced in presbyopia because of the low amplitude, relatively short line segments determine the base-in, phoria, and base-out lines. As a result, a small error can cause a relatively large distortion of the slope of the zone in presbyopia. One way to prevent this distortion is to perform near-point tests through more than one add and avoid adds that require the presbyope to use almost all the amplitude of accommodation. Another way to handle the problem is to use an alternative graph with the values of the accommodation and convergence scales spread out more.[18]

EXOPHORIA IN PRESBYOPIA

The high near-point exophoria often associated with presbyopic adds may or may not be associated with diplopia or asthenopic symptoms. Presbyopes with high near-point exophoria are less often symptomatic than are nonpresbyopes with comparable amounts of exophoria. This situation can be explained by the theory that presbyopes use more accommodative convergence at near to retain fusion.[19] They also tend to hold their work at a greater distance than young people and children do. When the exophoria does result in asthenopia, three alternatives are available for correction: (1) segments decentered to get a base-in effect (it may be necessary to use a wider segment when it is decentered so that the patient is not looking through the edge of the segment); (2) a separate prescription for near work, with base-in prism or decentering to obtain a base-in effect; and (3) base-out vision training. Orthoptic procedures to increase positive fusional convergence have a high success rate in presbyopia.[20-22]

Sheedy[23] emphasizes that fixation disparity should be evaluated when a large near-point exophoria is present. No correction may be necessary when an exo fixation disparity is not uncovered.

EXAMPLES

The individual depicted in Figure 12.2 has a working distance of 40 cm and an amplitude of accommodation of 3.50D. If half the amplitude is kept in reserve, the proper add is

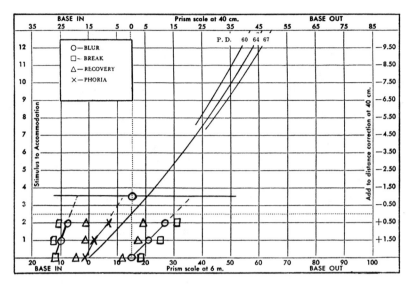

Figure 12.2 An example of findings in presbyopia.

	Phoria	Base-in	Base-out	Plus-to-Blur	Minus-to-Blur
6 m	1 exophoria	X/12/4	X/18/12		
40 cm + 0.50	8 exophoria	22/26/16	12/16/4	+2.00	−1.50
40 cm + 1.50	13 exophoria	25/28/16	6/10/2		

Amplitude of accommodation = 3.50D. Patient's working distance = approximately 40 cm.

Add = 2.50 − 3.50/2
    = 2.50 − 1.75
    = +0.75D

An add of +0.75D also would make the plus-to-blur finding equal to the minus-to-blur finding. If we determine where a +0.75 add will be on the graph, we can guess that the phoria will be approximately 9 exo and the base-out reserve will be approximately 11. Thus, Sheard's criterion will not be met with this add. If the fixation disparity or the symptoms warrant it, the corrective procedures for exophoria in presbyopia discussed earlier can be used.

A second example appears in Figure 12.3. With a working distance of 33 cm and an amplitude of 2.00D, keeping half the amplitude in reserve indicates an add of +2.00D:

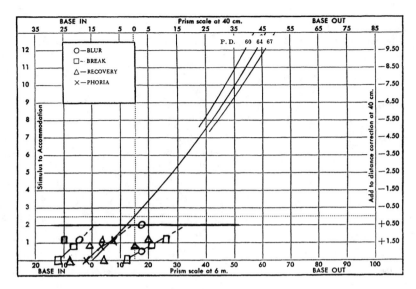

Figure 12.3 Another example of findings in presbyopia.

	Phoria	Base-in	Base-out	Plus-to-Blur	Minus-to-Blur
6 m	2 exophoria	X/12/8	X/12/4		
40 cm + 1.75	12 exophoria	X/22/16	X/6/0		
33 cm + 1.75	11 exophoria	24/28/14	X/8/2	+ 0.75	− 0.75

Amplitude of accommodation = 2.00D. Patient's working distance = 33 cm.

Add = 3.00D − 2.00D/2

    = +2.00D

The plus-to-blur and minus-to-blur findings are equal with a +1.75 add, so one would probably use a +1.75 or +2.00D add, depending largely on the patient's previous prescription and symptoms. Because of the high ACA ratio, the exophoria will probably be approximately 2Δ higher through the +2.00D add than through the +1.75D add. On this basis, the lower add may be preferable. Even with this lower add, however, Sheard's criterion is not met, so some corrective procedures may be necessary if the patient is symptomatic. Although there is a high exophoria at near through the add at this time, the particular patient may have been an esophore at near in the nonpresbyopic years. We can suggest this by extending the phoria line beyond the amplitude. If we do so, the phoria line will cross the 2.50D stimulus to accommodation level, for example, 5Δ to the right of the demand line.

Case Report: Patient GV

Patient GV, a 48-year-old male college professor, complained of near-point blur. He stated that he now had to hold reading material out farther than he would like to when wearing his glasses, but that he had to hold things too close without his glasses. His preferred reading distance was approximately 40 cm. His spectacles were 4 years old. Their powers were −2.25–0.50 × 5 OD, −3.00–0.25 × 175 OS, +1.00D add. Visual acuities with these spectacles were 6/4.5 OD, 6/4.5–1/6 OS, 6/4.5 OU at distance and 20/30 OD, 20/30 + 2/8 OS, 20/30 + 2/8 OU at near. The cover test with the current correction revealed orthophoria at distance and a slight exophoria at near. The subjective refraction findings were −2.50–0.25 × 165 OD (6/4.5), −3.00–0.50 × 160 OS (6/4.5). The distance dissociated phoria with these lenses was 1Δ esophoria. The distance fusional vergence ranges were base-in X/8/2, base-out 8/24/12. The near BCC test yielded a +1.50D add. The NRA and PRA starting from this add were +0.75D and −0.75D, respectively. Through the +1.50D add the dissociated phoria at 40 cm was zero. This patient had no distance vision complaint. This is consistent with the minimal change from the distance portion of the habitual prescription to the subjective refraction (the change in spherical equivalent was −0.12D for both OD and OS). The case history and the test findings suggest an increase in the plus add. Balancing the NRA and PRA suggests a +1.50D add over the subjective refraction. This is a change of +0.37D OD and OS in the spherical equivalent total near-point power from the habitual prescription. The patient reported that the subjective refraction lenses in a trial frame gave good distance vision and that the +1.50D add over that provided clear comfortable near vision. Progressive addition lenses with those powers were ordered.

Case Report: Patent JK

Patient JK, a 43-year-old female nurse, complained of some difficulty seeing fine print. She had spectacles that were several years old and that she wore them only to drive. These spectacles had powers of −0.50D sphere OD, −1.00 D sphere OS. Unaided visual acuities were 6/6 OD, 6/7.5 + 3/6 OS, 6/6 OU at distance, and 20/40–2/6 OD, 20/30–2/8 OS, 20/30 OU. The cover test without correction showed orthophoria at distance and near. The subjective refraction findings were plano sphere OD (6/6 + 2/6), −0.50 D sphere OS (6/6 + 3/6). The distance dissociated phoria with these lenses was 1Δ esophoria. The distance fusional vergence ranges were base-in X/12/4, base-out 18/24/4. The plus build-up indicated a minimum plus of +0.75 D add over the distance refractive correction to read 20/20 at 40 cm. The BCC result was a +1.50D add. The dissociated phoria and fusional vergence ranges at 40 cm through the +1.50D add from the BCC test were 4Δ exophoria; base-in 16/20/14, base-out 10/16/4. The NRA and PRA findings were +1.00D and −1.25D, respectively, over the BCC finding. Balancing the NRA and PRA suggests a plus add of +1.25D. This is a total near-point power of +1.25D OD, +0.75D OS. When JK looked at magazine print through these lenses in a trial frame, she reported that the print was easy to read. Progressive addition lenses with powers of plano sphere OD, −0.50D sphere OS, +1.25D add were ordered.

REFERENCES

1. Cline D, Hofstetter HW, Griffin JR. *Dictionary of Visual Science.* 4th ed. Radnor, PA: Chilton; 1989:551.
2. Cline D, Hofstetter HW, Griffin JR. *Dictionary of Visual Science.* 4th ed. Radnor, PA: Chilton; 1989:26–27.
3. Carlson NB, Kurtz D, Heath DA, Hines C. *Clinical Procedures for Ocular Examination.* Norwalk, CT: Appleton & Lange; 1990:11–12.
4. London R. Amplitude of accommodation. In: Eskridge JB, Amos JF, Bartlett JD, eds. *Clinical Procedures in Optometry.* Philadelphia, PA: Lippincott; 1991:69–71.
5. Hofstetter HW. A comparison of Duane's and Donders' tables of the amplitude of accommodation. *Am J Optom Arch Am Acad Optom.* 1944;21:345–363.
6. Hofstetter HW. A useful age-amplitude formula. *Pennsylvania Optom.* 1947;7:5–8.
7. Borish IM. *Clinical Refraction.* 3rd ed. Chicago, IL: Professional Press; 1970:178–184.
8. Patorgis CJ. Presbyopia. In: Amos JF. ed. *Diagnosis and Management in Vision Care.* Boston, MA: Butterworth-Heinemann; 1987:203–238.
9. Hanlon SD, Nakabayashi J, Shigezawa G. A critical view of presbyopic add determination. *J Am Optom Assoc.* 1987;58:468–472.
10. Grosvenor TP. *Primary Care Optometry.* 2nd ed. Boston, MA: Butterworth-Heinemann, 1989:334–336.
11. Fannin TE. Presbyopic addition. In: Eskridge JB, Amos JF, Bartlett JD, eds. *Clinical Procedures in Optometry.* Philadelphia, PA: Lippincott; 1991:198–205.
12. Hofstetter HW. A survey of practices in prescribing presbyopic adds. *Am J Optom Arch Am Acad Optom.* 1949;26:144–160.
13. Morgan MW. Accommodative changes in presbyopia and their correction. In: Hirsch MJ, Wick RE, eds. *Vision of the Aging Patient.* Philadelphia, PA: Chilton 1960:83–112.
14. Hofstetter HW. The accommodative range through the near correction. *Am J Optom Arch Am Acad Optom.* 1948;25:275–285.
15. Hofstetter HW. The zone of clear single binocular vision. *Am J Optom Arch Am Acad Optom.* 1945;22:301–333, 361–384.

16. Alpern M. Types of movement. In: Davson H, ed. *Muscular Mechanisms.* 2nd ed. Vol 3 of *The Eye.* New York, NY: Academic; 1969:65–174.
17. Fry GA. Basic concepts underlying graphical analysis. In: Schor CM, Ciuffreda KJ, eds. *Vergence Eye Movements: Basic and Clinical Aspects.* Boston, MA: Butterworth-Heinemann; 1983:403–437.
18. Abel CA, Hofstetter HW. *The Graphical Analysis of Clinical Optometric Findings.* Los Angeles, CA: Los Angeles College of Optometry; 1951:183–186.
19. Sheedy JE, Saladin JJ. Exophoria at near in presbyopia. *Am J Optom Physiol Opt.* 1975;52:474–481.
20. Vodnoy BE. Orthoptics for the advanced presbyope. *Optom Weekly.* 1975;66:204–206.
21. Wick B. Vision training for presbyopic nonstrabismic patients. *Am J Optom Physiol Opt.* 1977;54:244–247.
22. Cohen AH, Soden R. Effectiveness of visual therapy for convergence insufficiencies for an adult population. *J Am Optom Assoc.* 1984;55:491–494.
23. Sheedy JE. Analysis of near oculomotor balance. *Rev Optom.* 1979;116:44–45.

SUGGESTED READING

Fannin TE. Presbyopic addition. In: Eskridge JB, Amos JF, Bartlett JD, eds. *Clinical Procedures in Optometry.* Philadelphia, PA: Lippincott; 1991:198–205.
Grosvenor TP. *Primary Care Optometry.* 2nd ed. Boston, MA: Butterworth-Heinemann; 1989:334–336.
Morgan MW. Accommodative changes in presbyopia and their correction. In: Hirsch MJ, Wick RE, eds. *Vision of the Aging Patient.* Philadelphia, PA: Chilton; 1960:83–112.
Patorgis CJ. Presbyopia. In: Amos JF, ed. *Diagnosis and Management in Vision Care.* Boston, MA: Butterworth-Heinemann; 1987:203–238.

PRACTICE PROBLEMS

Graph the findings for the following patients and answer the questions:

1. What add would be given on the basis of the rule: Keep half the amplitude in reserve?

2. What add would be given on the basis of the balance of PRA and NRA at the working distance?

3. What is the ACA ratio?

4. Is Sheard's criterion met with the proposed add (a) at 40 cm? (b) at 33 cm? (c) at the working distance?

5. On the basis of the information available, what add, therapy, or prescription would you provide?

	Patient EB	**Patient TC**	**Patient JF**	**Patient CB**
Working distance	33 cm	36 cm	40 cm	40 cm
Amplitude of accommodation	2.00D	2.75D	3.00D	2.50D
6 m phoria	1 exophoria	orthophoria	1 esophoria	2 exophoria
6 m base-in limit	11 (break)	9 (break)	8 (break)	12 (break)
6 m base-out limit	14 (break)	13 (blur)	17 (blur)	12 (blur)
Add used below	+ 2.00	+ 1.25	+ 1.00	+ 1.00
40 cm phoria	14 exophoria	9 exophoria	1 esophoria	12 exophoria
40 cm base-in limit		18 (blur)	11 (blur)	23 (blur)
40 cm base-out limit		7 (blur)	16 (blur)	4 (blur)
40 cm plus-to-blur	+ 0.25	+ 1.00	+ 1.50	+ 1.00
40 cm minus-to-blur	− 1.50	− 1.50	− 1.50	− 1.00

	Patient EB	Patient TC	Patient JF	Patient CB
Add used below			+ 1.50	+ 1.50
40 cm phoria			5 exophoria	14 exophoria
40 cm base-in limit				
40 cm base-out limit				
40 cm plus-to-blur			+ 1.00	
40 cm minus-to-blur			− 2.00	
Add used below	+ 2.00	+ 1.25		
33 cm phoria	15 exophoria	10 exophoria		
33 cm base-in limit	27 (blur)	20 (blur)		
33 cm base-out limit	4 (break)	7 (break)		
33 cm plus-to-blur	+ 0.50	+ 1.25		
33 cm minus-to-blur	− 1.00	− 1.00		

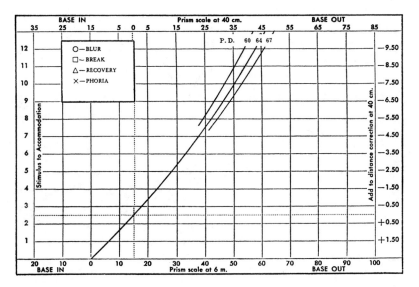

Patient EB

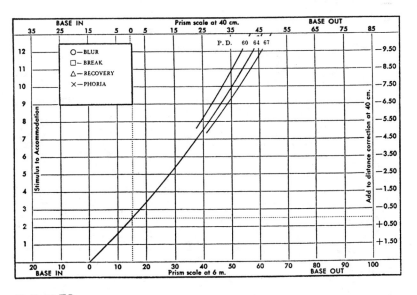

Patient TC

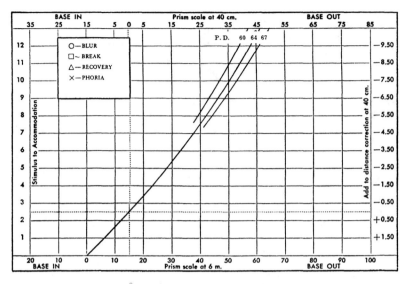

Patient JF

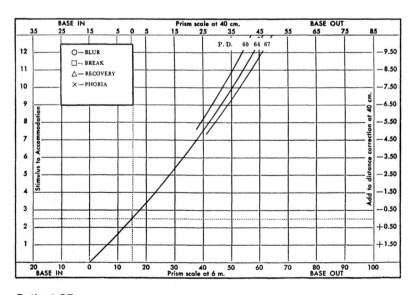

Patient CB

13

Nonpresbyopic Accommodative Disorders

Accommodative disorders in nonpresbyopic individuals can result in blurred vision, headaches, ocular discomfort, and/or other difficulties associated with near work. Accommodative dysfunction in nonpresbyopes is relatively common.[1,2] The treatments for nonpresbyopic accommodative disorders, plus lens adds and vision training, are very effective in relieving ocular symptoms.[1,3-7] Probably the best first step toward an understanding of nonpresbyopic accommodative disorders is to understand the tests used in evaluating accommodative function.

TESTS OF ACCOMMODATIVE FUNCTION

Clinical tests of accommodative function can be grouped into four categories: (1) amplitude of accommodation, (2) accommodative facility, (3) tests that directly or indirectly assess lag of accommodation, and (4) relative accommodation. Amplitude of accommodation is a measure of the maximum amount of accommodation an individual can exert. As discussed in Chapter 12, amplitude of accommodation usually is determined by the push-up test.[8,9]

Tests for accommodative facility examine the speed of accommodative changes.[10,11] The dioptric accommodative stimulus is alternated between two different levels. The patient reports when a letter target first is seen clearly after each alternation in accommodative stimulus. The examiner counts the number of cycles completed in 1 minute (one cycle being the change from one stimulus level to the other and back again). Accommodative stimulus can be varied either by lens power changes or by viewing distance changes. The former often is referred to as "lens rock" and the latter as "distance rock," indicating that the accommodative stimulus level is "rocked" back and forth.

The standard method of testing accommodative facility is a lens rock procedure using a pair of +2.00D lenses on one side of a flipper bar and −2.00D lenses on the other side (Figure 13.1). The test is begun with the +2.00D lenses over the patient's refractive correction. A test

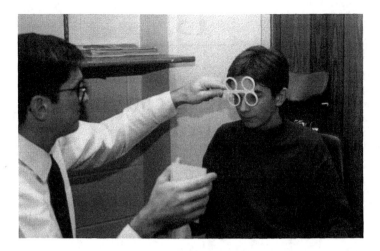

Figure 13.1 Lens rock accommodative facility testing with a flipper bar. The patient views letters on a near-point card. Each time the patient reports clarity of the letters, the lens bar is flipped to place the lenses of opposite sign power in front of the patient's eyes. An accommodative facility rate in cycles per minute is recorded. One cycle is a change from plus to minus to plus.

distance of 40 cm usually is used with reduced Snellen letters at a 20/20 to 20/30 acuity demand. The patient is asked to report each time the letters first appear clear after each flip of the lens bar. The number of cycles per minute is recorded.

Clinically measured lens rock accommodative facility rates correlate with objectively measured latency periods and velocities of change in accommodative response.[4,12] Children with ocular symptoms have been reported to have lower lens rock facility rates than asymptomatic children.[13] The mean flipper rates reported in different studies show quite a bit of variability.[13–18] Cut-offs for test failure used by many clinicians using +2.00D/−2.00D flippers and a 40-cm viewing distance for children and adults up to approximately 30 years of age are less than 11 cycles per minute for monocular testing[13,16,19,20] and less than 8 cycles per minute for binocular testing.[13,19,21]

Accommodative facility rates are greater if larger letters, lower-power lenses, or a closer test distance is used.[22] Therefore, it is important that the examiner maintain a consistent testing technique. Accommodative facility testing is associated with strong practice effects.[19,21] Rouse et al[21] have thus recommended that if a failing rate is found in a 1-minute testing period, testing should be repeated for a second and a third minute. Test failure is indicated if the rates remain below the cut-off for test failure or decline over the second and third minutes of testing.

During binocular lens rock testing, adjustments in fusional vergence must occur to compensate for changes in accommodative vergence. Therefore, patients may pass the monocular lens rock but fail the binocular lens rock if a vergence disorder is present. Some clinicians have emphasized using a vectographic target for binocular lens rock facility to control for suppression.[23–25]

Haynes[26] has described a distance rock accommodative facility test procedure. Rocking between 20/20 letters at 6 m, 20/25 letters at 6 m, and 20/25 letters at 40 cm, a sample of students and clinic patients ranging in age from 18 to 35 years averaged 25 cycles per minute.[26] Distance rock rates are higher than lens rock rates.[18] Additional testing will be necessary to establish normative values for distance rock accommodative facility.

The third category of accommodation tests includes tests that directly or indirectly assess the patient's lag of accommodation.[27] During accommodation for near-point viewing, the retina usually is conjugate with a point slightly behind the object of regard. In other words, for near-point targets, accommodative response usually is slightly less than the accommodative stimulus.[28,29] The amount by which the dioptric accommodative response is less than the dioptric accommodative stimulus is the lag of accommodation. The uncommon situation in which the accommodative response is greater than the accommodative stimulus is known as a "lead of accommodation."

The third category of accommodation tests can be further divided into (1) tests that measure the lag of accommodation and (2) tests in which lens power is changed to alter accommodative stimulus to the point at which dioptric accommodative stimulus and dioptric accommodative response are equal.[11] Examples of the former are monocular estimation method (MEM) dynamic retinoscopy and Nott dynamic retinoscopy. Examples of the latter are low neutral dynamic retinoscopy and the binocular cross-cylinder (BCC) test.

A test card with an aperture in the center usually is used for dynamic retinoscopy so that the examiner can observe the retinoscopic reflex close to the patient's visual axis through the aperture (Figure 13.2).[30] In MEM dynamic retinoscopy the amount of the lag of accommodation is estimated by judging the width, speed, and brightness of the retinoscopic reflex.[1,31,32] The test card and the retinoscope are placed at the same distance from the patient's spectacle plane, usually 40 cm. The patient's distance refractive correction is placed in a trial frame or the phoropter. With the retinoscope in plane mirror mode, with motion indicates a lag of accommodation and against motion indicates a lead of accommodation. Neutrality indicates that accommodative stimulus and accommodative response are equal. The examiner's estimate of the amount of plus power that would be required to neutralize

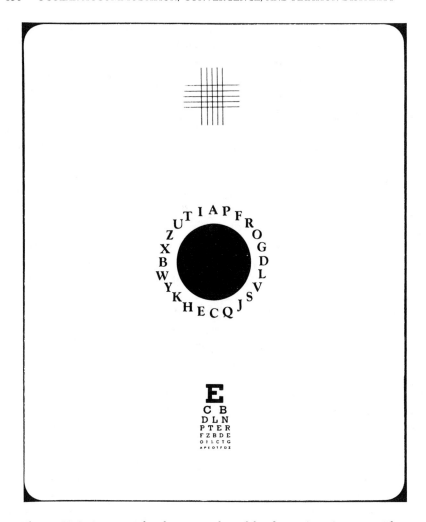

Figure 13.2 An example of a test card used for dynamic retinoscopy. The patient is directed to look at the letters just outside the aperture in the card. The examiner observes the retinoscopic reflex through the aperture in the card.

the with motion is the estimate of the lag of accommodation. The estimate of the lag can be confirmed by very briefly placing a plus lens equal in power to the estimated lag over one eye and quickly checking to see whether neutrality is observed. The lens should only be in place a half second or less so that a change in accommodative response is not induced.

Rouse et al[33] found that MEM dynamic retinoscopy results correlate very closely with subjective optometer measurements of accommodation. In another study, Rouse et al[34] reported a mean lag of 0.34D in school children using MEM dynamic retinoscopy. Jackson and Goss[18] reported a mean lag of 0.23D with MEM in school children. Most nonpresbyopic patients have lags of 0 to 0.75D with MEM retinoscopy.

Nott[35] is credited with the development of a form of dynamic retinoscopy in which the lag of accommodation is measured by moving the retinoscope behind the plane of the test card. The test card usually is suspended from the phoropter reading rod rather than attached to the retinoscope. The patient views the test card, usually placed at 40 cm from the spectacle plane, through the distance refractive correction. A with motion observed by the examiner indicates a lag of accommodation. The examiner moves back away from the patient slowly until a neutral retinoscopic reflex is seen.[27] The dioptric accommodative stimulus is the reciprocal of the test distance in meters. If the card is at 40 cm from the spectacle plane, the accommodative stimulus is 2.50D. The dioptric accommodative response is the reciprocal of the distance of the retinoscope from the spectacle plane in meters when neutral is observed. If neutral is noted with the retinoscope 50 cm from the spectacle plane, the accommodative response is 2.00D. In this case the lag of accommodation would be 0.50D. Jackson and Goss[18] reported a mean lag of 0.21D for a sample of children between the ages of 7 and 15 years.

Low neutral dynamic retinoscopy yields the lens power with which the dioptric accommodative stimulus and dioptric accommodative response are equal.[11,36] The retinoscope and the test card are maintained at the same distance from the patient, usually 40 cm from the spectacle plane. Testing is started with the patient's distance refractive correction in place. If a lag is observed, plus lenses are added in 0.25D steps until a neutral retinoscopic reflex is observed. The lens power added for neutrality is recorded. If, for example, the test result is +0.75D with a 40 cm distance, then the accommodative stimulus is 0.75D less than the 2.50D for the test distance, or 1.75D. Since neutral was observed at that point, the accommodative response is also 1.75D.

Cross[36,37] may have been the first to advocate adding lenses as a part of dynamic retinoscopy testing, so this is sometimes referred to as "Cross dynamic retinoscopy." Sheard proposed adding plus to the first neutral, the so-called low neutral point, as the end-point of testing.[38,39] Average values reported in the literature for low neutral dynamic retinoscopy have varied from +0.25 to +0.75D.[18,36,40]

The BCC test also yields a lens power with which dioptric accommodative stimulus and dioptric accommodative response are equal.[11,41,42] The BCC test differs from low neutral dynamic retinoscopy in that verbal responses are required from the patient, and in that the test is started with plus over the distance subjective refraction and plus is reduced to the test end-point. Details of testing procedure have been described by various authors.[43–45]

The relative accommodative tests are the plus-to-blur (or negative relative accommodation [NRA]) and the minus-to-blur (or positive relative accommodation [PRA]) tests.[46,47] The plotting of these tests in the zone of clear single binocular vision (ZCSBV) was discussed in Chapter 3. The NRA test often is limited by the positive fusional vergence capabilities of the patient, in which case it is plotted on the right side of the ZCSBV. The PRA usually is found on the top of the ZCSBV, in which case the amplitude of accommodation is the limiting factor, or the left side of the ZCSBV, indicating that the negative fusional vergence is the limiting factor. If the NRA or PRA points are inside the boundaries of the ZCSBV, there may have been a procedural error or the patient may have a deficit in optical reflex accommodation.

COMPARISONS OF ACCOMMODATION TESTS

Wick and Hall[48] performed tests of accommodative lag, facility, and amplitude during a vision screening of schoolchildren, and found that failure on one of these tests did not effectively predict failure on the other two tests.

Locke and Somers[49] compared MEM retinoscopy, low neutral dynamic retinoscopy, bell retinoscopy (another form of dynamic retinoscopy), and the BCC test using two examiners and 10 young subjects. They reported that the two examiners found values that were not significantly different on the four tests. Findings obtained with MEM, low neutral, and bell dynamic retinoscopy were not significantly different from each other, but they did differ from findings obtained using the BCC test.

Jackson and Goss[18] compared the results of several accommodation tests in 244 schoolchildren. The tests included MEM, low neutral, and Nott dynamic retinoscopy and NRA, PRA, BCC, lens rock, and distance rock tests. The lens rock and distance rock accommodative facility tests correlated significantly with each other, but generally not significantly or highly with other tests. The monocular estimation method, Nott and low neutral retinoscopy and the BCC showed significant correlations with each other, but not with most other tests.

The above three studies suggest that a complete work-up of accommodative function should include tests from each of the four test type categories discussed earlier in the chapter. In other words, a complete investigation of accommodative function should include (1) amplitude of accommodation, (2) accommodative facility, (3) NRA and PRA, and (4) some form of dynamic retinoscopy and/or the BCC test.

PRESCRIPTION AND MANAGEMENT GUIDELINES

Common symptoms of accommodative disorders are blur, eye strain, and headaches. The push-up amplitude of accommodation can be compared with the range of amplitudes expected for the patient's age based on Hofstetter's formulas given in the previous chapter. If the measured push-up amplitude is less than the minimum expected, then a plus add may be indicated.[1,50–52] If no organic factor can be recognized as the cause of the reduced amplitude, then vision training may be used to try to improve accommodative function.[1,50–52] If the amplitude of accommodation declines on repeated testing, vision training or a plus add also may be used.

The most common symptoms of poor accommodative facility are transient near-point blur and distance blur after near-point viewing. The treatment for poor accommodative facility is vision training procedures to improve facility.[51,52] These procedures are usually referred to as "accommodative rock." Accommodative rock training has been shown to be successful in increasing facility rates, in improving accommodative latencies and velocities, and in relieving ocular symptoms.[4–7,12,53]

A plus add may be indicated if the PRA is low. Finding the lens power that balances the NRA and PRA is a way of prescribing plus adds for nonpresbyopes,[54] just as for presbyopes, as discussed in the previous chapter.

The treatment of choice for a high lag of accommodation is a plus add.[51,52] If the lag of accommodation as determined by MEM or Nott retinoscopy is greater then 0.75D, one way of prescribing an add is to deduct 0.25D from the lag. If the plus added for neutrality on low neutral dynamic retinoscopy is greater than 1.00D, one way of determining the add is to deduct 0.50D from the test end-point. Allowing the patient to look at reading material with the proposed add in a trial frame is useful as a subjective evaluation of the add and as a demonstration to the patient. Vision training designed to improve the accommodative response also can be used in high-lag cases. A lead of accommodation is managed by vision training techniques designed to train reduction in accommodative response. A lead of accommodation may be secondary to a high exophoria. A lead sometimes occurs in exophoria because accommodative convergence is used to maintain fusion. If this is the case, the vision training program should include training to improve positive fusional vergence.

TERMS USED FOR ACCOMMODATIVE DISORDERS

There are some terms in common usage for accommodative disorders, although there is some variation in how they are defined.[1,51,52,55,56] "Accommodative insufficiency" is an abnormally low amplitude of accommodation. We can include a high lag of accommodation as part of accommodative insufficiency. A total lack of accommodation is called "paralysis of accommodation." Paralysis of accommodation is a rare condition that is caused by ocular disease or trauma. A reduction in the amplitude of accommodation with repeated testing is "accommodative fatigue." Poor accommodative facility is called "accommodative infacility." The condition in which a lead of accommodation exists is sometimes referred to as "accommodative excess." The typical examination findings and the treatment of choice for the most common accommodative disorders are given in Table 13.1.

Case Report: Patient MS

Patient MS, a 21-year-old female college student, complained of distance blur and headaches after reading. She had worn glasses for her distance vision before, but had lost them. Unaided visual acuities were 6/7.5 OD, OS, OU at distance and 20/20 OD, OS, OU at near. The cover test showed orthophoria at distance and exophoria at near. The subjective refraction was −0.50 D sphere OD (6/4.5), −0.50-0.25 × 180 OS (6/4.5). Some of the examination findings are shown in Figure 13.3. The phoria findings suggest convergence insufficiency. However, the fact that the phoria line does not tilt to the right as far as the left and right sides of the ZCSBV suggests pseudoconvergence insufficiency. In addition, the slightly low amplitude of accommodation for her age and the higher plus value on the BCC test suggest accommodative insufficiency. Other findings confirming the pseudo-convergence insufficiency form of accommodative insufficiency were that (1) the near-point of convergence improved from 9 cm with no lenses in place to 7 cm with +0.50D lenses in front of each eye (on repeated testing the near-point of convergence results were 9.5 cm with no lenses and 7 cm with +0.50D lenses), and (2) with no lenses in place the lag of accommodation with Nott dynamic retinoscopy was 0.94D. The patient reported that −0.50D lenses in a trial frame improved distance vision and +0.50D lenses made magazine print

Table 13.1
Summary of test findings and recommended treatment for the most common non-presbyopic accommodative disorders.

	Amplitude of Accommodation	Accommodative Facility	Lag of Accommodation	Relative Accommodation	Other Findings	Treatment of Choice
Accommodative insufficiency	low for age	may be slow on minus side of flippers, slow coming in on distance rock	high	NRA normal, PRA low	sometimes pseudoconvergence insufficiency	plus add with power derived from dynamic retinoscopy and confirmed by subjective evaluation by the patient
Accommodative infacility	normal	poor	normal	both NRA and PRA may be low	transient blur a very common complaint	vision training to improve accommodative facility
Accommodative fatigue	normal initially; declines with repeated testing	normal initially; may decrease with continued testing	normal initially; may high after prolonged near work	PRA normal or low		vision training or plus add
Accommodative excess	normal	may be slow on plus side of flippers, slow going out on distance rock	lead of accommodation	NRA normal or low	sometimes high exophoria	vision training to relax accommodation; if high exophoria present, also training to improve positive fusional vergence

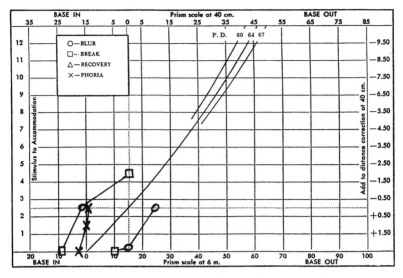

Figure 13.3 Test results and ZCSBV for patient MS.

	Phoria	Base-in	Base-out	Plus-to-Blur	Minus-to-Blur
6 m	2 exophoria	X/9/4	X/10/4		
40 cm	14 exophoria	16/24/16	10/12/4	+2.25	−2.00 (break)
40 cm +1.00	15 exophoria				

Amplitude of accommodation = 9D; BCC test = +1.50D.

appear easier to read. The prescription given the patient was −0.50D sphere OD, −0.50–0.25 × 180 OS, +1.00D add in progressive addition lenses.

Case Report: Patient MP

Patient MP, a 21-year-old male college student, complained of distance blur after near work and occasional blur at near. His spectacles were about 1 year 6 months old, and they had powers of −0.50–0.50 × 105 OD, −0.50–0.50 × 60 OS. His distance visual acuities with this correction were 6/6–2/6 OD, 6/6–1/6 OS, 6/6–1/6 OU, and near acuities were 20/20–1/8 OD, OS, OU. It appeared that orthophoria was

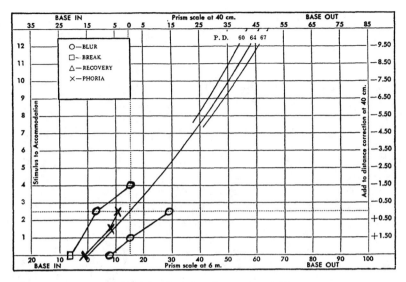

Figure 13.4 Test findings and ZCSBV for patient MP.

	Phoria	Base-in	Base-out	Plus-to-Blur	Minus-to-Blur
6 m	1 exophoria	X/7/4	8/14/12		
40 cm	4 exophoria	12/14/9	14/18/10	+1.50	−1.50
40 cm +1.00	7 exophoria				

PD = 64 mm.

present at distance and a slight exophoria at near when the cover test was performed with the habitual spectacles. The subjective refraction was −0.75–0.50 × 105 OD (6/4.5), −0.75–0.50 × 75 OS (6/4.5). Some of the examination findings and the ZCSBV are given in Figure 13.4. The patient's chief complaint suggested accommodative infacility. This was confirmed by flipper testing. He could not clear either side of the +2.00/−2.00D flippers. He achieved only six cycles per minute with +1.50/−1.50D flippers. He was instructed in accommodative facility exercises to be done at home on a daily basis. He also was scheduled for weekly clinic visits for additional training and follow-up checks. At the end of a 4-week training program his NRA and PRA had increased to +2.50 and −3.00 D, respectively, and he had a binocular accommodative facility rate of 10 cycles per minute on +2.00/−2.00D flippers. He reported that he no longer had occasional blurring and that he could read for up to 2 hours without his eyes getting tired.

REFERENCES

1. Daum KM. Accommodative dysfunction. *Doc Ophthalmol.* 1983;55:177–198.
2. Hokoda SC. General binocular dysfunctions in an urban optometry clinic. *J Am Optom Assoc.* 1985;56:560–562.
3. Wold RM, Pierce JR, Keddington J. Effectiveness of optometric vision therapy. *J Am Optom Assoc.* 1970;49:1047–1054.
4. Lui JS, Lee M, Jang J, et al. Objective assessment of accommodation orthoptics. I. Dynamic insufficiency. *Am J Optom Physiol Opt.* 1979;56:285–294.
5. Suchoff IB, Petito GT. The efficacy of visual therapy accommodative disorders and non-strabismic anomalies of binocular vision. *J Am Optom Assoc.* 1986;57:119–125.
6. Rouse MW. Management of binocular anomalies: efficacy of vision therapy in the treatment of accommodative disorders. *Am J Optom Physiol Opt.* 1987;64:415–420.
7. Cooper J, Feldman K, Selenow A, et al. Reduction of asthenopia after accommodative facility training. *Am J Optom Physiol Opt.* 1987;64:430–436.
8. Grosvenor TP. *Primary Care Optometry.* 2nd ed. Boston, MA: Butterworth-Heinemann; 1989:140–149.
9. London R. Amplitude of accommodation. In: Eskridge JB, Amos JF, Bartlett JD, eds. *Clinical Procedures in Optometry.* Philadelphia, PA: Lippincott; 1991:69–71.
10. Daum KM. Accommodative facility. In: Eskridge JB, Amos JF, Bartlett JD, eds. *Clinical Procedures in Optometry.* Philadelphia, PA: Lippincott; 1991:687–697.
11. Goss DA. Clinical accommodation testing. *Curr Opin Ophthalmol.* 1992;3:78–82.
12. Bobier WR, Sivak JG. Orthoptic treatment of subjects showing slow accommodative responses. *Am J Optom Physiol Opt.* 1983;60:678–687.
13. Hennessey D, Iosue RA, Rouse MW. Relation of symptoms to accommodative infacility of school-aged children. *Am J Optom Physiol Opt.* 1984;61:177–183.
14. Garzia P, Richman J. Accommodative facility: a study of young adults. *J Am Optom Assoc.* 1982;53:821–825.
15. Zellers JA, Albert TL, Rouse MW. A review of the literature and a normative study of accommodative facility. *J Am Optom Assoc.* 1984;55:31–37.
16. Levine S, Ciuffreda KJ, Selenow A, Flax N. Clinical assessment of accommodative facility in symptomatic and asymptomatic individuals. *J Am Optom Assoc.* 1985;56:286–290.
17. Scheiman M, Herberg H, Frantz K, Margolies M. Normative study of accommodative facility in elementary schoolchildren. *Am J Optom Physiol Opt.* 1988;65:127–134.
18. Jackson TW, Goss DA. Variation and correlation of clinical tests of accommodative function in a sample of school-age children. *J Am Optom Assoc.* 1991;62:857–866.
19. McKenzie KM, Kerr SR, Rouse MW, DeLand PN. Study of accommodative facility testing reliability. *Am J Optom Physiol Opt.* 1987;64:186–194.

20. Rouse MW, DeLand PN, Chous R, Determan TF. Monocular accommodative facility testing reliability. *Optom Vis Sci.* 1989;66:72–77.

21. Rouse MW, DeLand PN, Mozayani S, Smith JP. Binocular accommodative facility testing reliability. *Optom Vis Sci.* 1992;69:314–319.

22. Siderov J, Johnston AW. The importance of the test parameters in the clinical assessment of accommodative facility. *Optom Vis Sci.* 1990;67:551–557.

23. Pierce JR, Greenspan SB. Accommodative rock procedures in VT—a clinical guide. Part II. *Optom Weekly.* 1971;62:776–780.

24. Burge S. Suppression during binocular accommodative rock. *Optom Monthly.* 1979;79:867–872.

25. Scheiman M, Wick B. *Clinical Management of Binocular Vision—Heterophoric, Accommodative, and Eye Movement Disorders.* Philadelphia, PA: Lippincott; 1994:22–24.

26. Haynes HM. The distance rock test—a preliminary report. *J Am Optom Assoc.* 1979;50:707–713.

27. Daum KM. Accommodative response. In: Eskridge JB, Amos JF, Bartlett JD, eds. *Clinical Procedures in Optometry.* Philadelphia, PA: Lippincott; 1991: 677–686.

28. Ciuffreda KJ, Kenyon RV. Accommodative vergence and accommodation in normals, amblyopes, and strabismics. In: Schor CM, Ciuffreda KJ, eds. *Vergence Eye Movements: Basic and Clinical Aspects.* Boston, MA: Butterworth-Heinemann; 1983:101–173.

29. Ciuffreda KJ. Accommodation and its anomalies. In: Charman WN, ed. *Visual Optics and Instrumentation.* Boca Raton, FL: CRC Press; 1991:231–279.

30. Haynes HM. Clinical observations with dynamic retinoscopy. *Optom Weekly.* 1960;51:2243–2246, 2306–2309.

31. Bieber JC. Why nearpoint retinoscopy with children? *Optom Weekly.* 1974;65:54–57, 78–82.

32. Grosvenor TP. *Primary Care Optometry.* 2nd ed. Boston, MA: Butterworth-Heinemann, 1989:253–254.

33. Rouse MW, London R, Allen DC. An evaluation of the monocular estimate of dynamic retinoscopy. *Am J Optom Physiol Opt.* 1982;59:234–239.

34. Rouse MW, Hutter RF, Shiftlett R. A normative study of the accommodative lag in elementary school children. *Am J Optom Physiol Opt.* 1984;61: 693–697.

35. Nott IS. Dynamic skiametry, accommodation and convergence. *Am J Physiol Opt.* 1925;6:490–503.

36. Borish IM. *Clinical Refraction.* 3rd ed. Boston, MA: Butterworth-Heinemann; 1970:697–704.

37. Cross AJ. *Dynamic Skiametry in Theory and Practice.* New York, NY: Cross Optical Co; 1911:115–123.

38. Sheard C. Dynamic skiametry and methods of testing the accommodation and vergence of the eyes. In: *The Sheard Volume—Selected Writings in Visual and Ophthalmic Optics.* Philadelphia, PA: Chilton; 1957:125–230 (originally published as a monograph in 1920).

39. Guyton DL, O'Connor GM. Dynamic retinoscopy. *Curr Opin Ophthalmol.* 1991;2:78–80.

40. Haynes HM. Clinical approaches to nearpoint power determination. *Am J Optom Physiol Opt.* 1985;62:375–385.

41. Fry GA. Significance of fused cross cylinder test. *Optom Weekly.* 1940;31:16–19.

42. Goodson RA, Afanador AJ. The accommodative response to the near point crossed cylinder test. *Optom Weekly.* 1974;65:1138–1140.

43. Manas L. *Visual Analysis.* 3rd ed. Chicago, IL: Professional Press, 1965:154–156.

44. Borish IM. *Clinical Refraction.* 3rd ed. Boston, MA: Butterworth-Heinemann; 1970:839–842.

45. Grosvenor TP. *Primary Care Optometry.* 2nd ed. Boston, MA: Butterworth-Heinemann; 1989:288–290.

46. Grosvenor TP. *Primary Care Optometry.* 2nd ed. Boston, MA: Butterworth-Heinemann; 1989:291–292.

47. Carlson NB, Kurtz D, Heath DA, Hines C. *Clinical Procedures for Ocular Examination.* Norwalk, CT: Appleton & Lange; 1990:133–134.

48. Wick B, Hall P. Relation between accommodative facility, lag, and amplitude in elementary school children. *Am J Optom Physiol Opt.* 1987;64:593–598.

49. Locke LC, Somers W. A comparison study of dynamic retinoscopy techniques. *Optom Vis Sci.* 1989;66:540–544.

50. Daum K. Accommodative insufficiency. *Am J Optom Physiol Opt.* 1983;60: 352–359.

51. Cooper J. Accommodative dysfunction. In: Amos JF, ed. *Diagnosis and Management in Vision Care.* Boston, MA: Butterworth- Heinemann; 1987: 431–459.

52. Scheiman M, Wick B. *Clinical Management of Binocular Vision—Heterophoric, Accommodative, and Eye Movement Disorders.* Philadelphia, PA: Lippincott; 1994: 339–378.

53. Siderov J. Improving interactive facility with vision training. *Clinical and Experimental Optometry* 1990;73:128–131.

54. Birnbaum MH. *Optometric Management of Nearpoint Vision Disorders.* Boston, MA: Butterworth-Heinemann; 1993:161–167.

55. Duke-Elder S, Abrams D. *Ophthalmic Optics and Refraction.* Vol 5 in: Duke-Elder S, ed. *System of Ophthalmology.* St Louis, MO: Mosby; 1970:451–474.

56. Somers W, Locke LC. Accommodation terminology. *Optom Vis Sci.* 1990; 67:386. Reply.

SUGGESTED READING

Cooper J. Accommodative dysfunction. In: Amos JF, ed. *Diagnosis and Management in Vision Care.* Boston, MA: Butterworth; 1987:431–459.

Daum KM. Accommodative response. In: Eskridge JB, Amos JF, Bartlett JD, eds. *Clinical Procedures in Optometry.* Philadelphia, PA: Lippincott; 1991:677–686.

Daum KM. Accommodative facility. In: Eskridge JB, Amos JF, Bartlett JD, eds. *Clinical Procedures in Optometry.* 1991:687–697.

PRACTICE PROBLEMS

1. A 20-year-old patient has a push-up amplitude of accommodation of 7.00D. How does this compare to the minimum expected amplitude? What is the term applied to this condition? What are the potential treatments?

2. Nott retinoscopy was performed on three patients. The test distance was 40 cm. Neutrality was observed with the retinoscope at the following distances: patient CD, 48 cm; patient GI, 68 cm; and patient FC, 56 cm. In each case, what are the accommodative response and the lag of accommodation? Would treatment be indicated? If so, what treatment?

3. On MEM retinoscopy you estimate that you are approximately +1.25D away from neutrality. What is the lag of accommodation? Is this a normal or high lag?

4. Which of the two forms of accommodative facility testing includes both proximal and optical cues to the change in accommodative stimulus and which includes only optical cues? Explain.

14

Introduction to Vision Training for Accommodation and Convergence Disorders

Vision training can be used to increase positive fusional vergence (positive width of the zone of clear single binocular vision [ZCSBV]) and negative fusional vergence (negative width of the ZCSBV). If a low amplitude of accommodation is not due to disease, pharmacologic cause, or the normal aging process, vision training may be able to increase the amplitude of accommodation (height of the ZCSBV). Latency and velocity of accommodative and/or convergence responses also can be improved with vision training. This chapter will provide an introduction to some common simple vision training techniques for the improvement of accommodation and convergence function. Additional details on these and other training techniques can be found in texts devoted largely to vision training.[1-5]

Several investigators[6-10] have described the plotting of accommodation and convergence data to aid in understanding and designing vision training programs. The discussions below will use graphs to show how accommodation and convergence stimuli are changed in various training techniques. In each case a PD of 64 mm will be used, and it will be assumed that the patient's refractive correction is being worn. Lines and arrows on each graph show changes in accommodation and convergence stimuli induced by the training techniques. When used in the treatment of nonstrabismic accommodation or vergence disorders, these techniques are used daily in treatment programs that usually last for 3 to 6 weeks in duration.

PUSH-UP TRAINING

Push-up training is a common technique used to improve positive fusional convergence and the near-point of convergence. The patient brings a convenient fixation object closer in the mid-line until it feels as

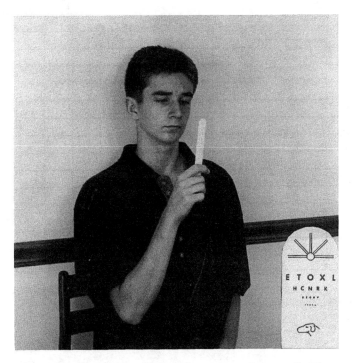

Figure 14.1 Push-up training. The patient tries to maintain singleness of the fixation object as it is brought closer. Various targets can be used for push-up training, such as letter targets affixed to a tongue depressor, as shown here. The target used here is shown in the lower right. The addition of small letters and features aids control of accommodation.

if the object will break into two or until it does (Figure 14.1). This is repeated several times so that the patient is able to bring the object closer before diplopia occurs. If small letters are included in the fixation object for better control of accommodation, this technique also can be used to improve the amplitude of accommodation when indicated. There is no built-in suppression control with this method. That is, there is no obvious way to make the patient aware of suppression if it is occurring. One way to check for suppression is to have the patient be aware of physiologic diplopia occasionally during the push-up training.

Since the convergence stimulus and the accommodative stimulus are varied by changing target distance, changes in convergence and accommodative stimuli can be represented on the graph by movement along the demand line. For example, Figure 14.2 shows the change in stimulus levels when a object is moved from 25 cm in to 10 cm away from the spectacle plane.

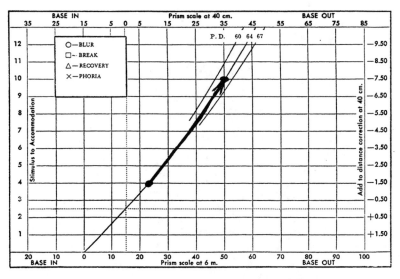

Figure 14.2 Example of the changes in convergence and accommodative stimuli during push-up training with the fixation object moved from 25 cm in to 10 cm away.

BROCK STRING

The Brock string (Figure 14.3) provides a simple, but very useful and versatile, training technique. One end of the string is tied to a chair, door knob, or other object, while the other end is held against the nose. The patient is instructed to maintain singleness of the bead being fixated. The bead is moved closer to the patient for push-up training or farther from the patient for push-away training. Vergence facility can be improved by having the patient alternate fixation between two or more beads.

One advantage of the Brock string is that it provides obvious suppression controls. The string should appear to be an X crossing at the fixated bead, due to physiologic diplopia. Also as a consequence of physiologic diplopia, the beads not being fixated should appear doubled. One way in which the Brock string is versatile is that it can be used for training in different fields of gaze.

An example of the accommodative and convergence stimuli in vergence facility training with the Brock string is shown in Figure 14.4. If the patient alternates fixation between beads at 1 m and 12.5 cm, the accommodative and convergence stimuli would change back and forth between the levels represented by the 1-m and 12.5-cm demand line points. Another way in which the Brock string is versatile is that the convergence and accommodative stimuli also can be adjusted by training with spherical lens adds or prisms, such as with lens or prism flippers.

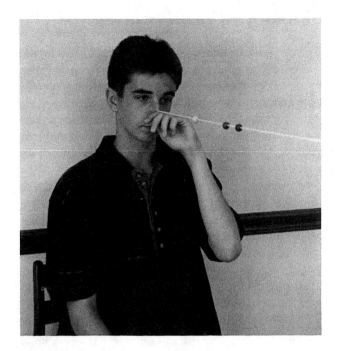

Figure 14.3 Brock string training.

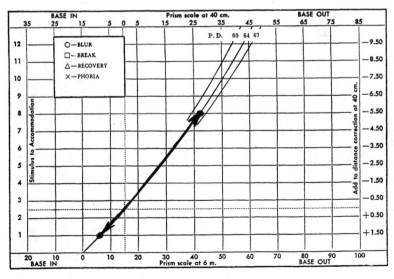

Figure 14.4 Example of the changes in accommodative and convergence stimuli during Brock string training with the patient alternating fixation between beads at 1 m and 12.5 cm.

VECTOGRAMS AND TRANAGLYPHS

Vectograms are polarized targets in which one is seen by the right eye and one by the left eye when polarized goggles are worn (Figure 14.5). Tranaglyphs are anaglyph targets in which one target is seen by the right eye and one by the left eye when a red filter is worn over one eye and a green filter over the other. Vectograms and tranaglyphs are used to train positive fusional convergence and negative fusional convergence. Points of similarity on the targets are fused, while points of dissimilarity are used as clues that suppression is occurring.

A base-out stimulus can be induced by moving the target seen by the left eye to the right of the target seen by the right eye. The lines of sight thus cross between the patient and the target. If the patient's spectacle plane is 40 cm from the vectogram and the targets are slowly separated to increase the base-out stimulus from 0 (no target separation) to 20Δ base-out, the change in accommodation and convergence would be as illustrated in Figure 14.6. Note that the accommodative stimulus is unchanged, so only positive fusional convergence is stimulated.

A base-in stimulus is induced if the target seen by the left eye is moved to the left of the target seen by the right eye. Therefore, the lines of sight

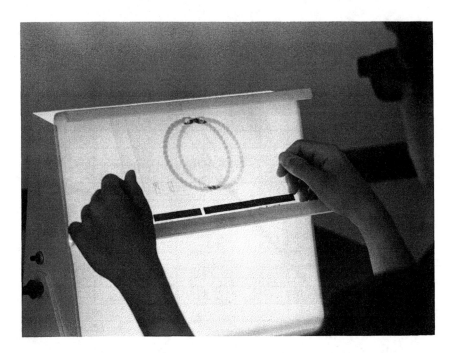

Figure 14.5 A vectogram from Bernell Corporation. One of the targets is seen by the right eye and one by the left eye when polaroid goggles are worn.

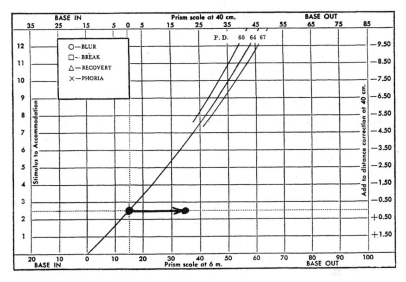

Figure 14.6 Example of the change in convergence stimulus when base-out training is done with a vectogram.

of the two eyes cross behind the plane of the target. This stimulates negative fusional convergence. If the convergence stimulus from target separation is changed from 0 to 10 base-in, the total convergence stimulus would change from 15Δ (target distance = 40 cm) to 5Δ (Figure 14.7).

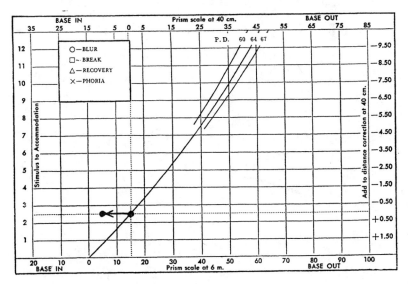

Figure 14.7 Example of the change in convergence stimulus when base-in training is done with a vectogram.

BINOCULAR LENS ROCK

Binocular lens rock is a technique used to improve accommodative facility. A pair of plus lenses and a pair of minus lenses (usually +2.00 and −2.00D, but may be lower powers at the start of a training program) in a lens flipper bar are used to vary the accommodative stimulus. This training procedure is done in the same way that lens rock accommodative facility testing is done (see Figure 13.1).

The plus lenses decrease the accommodative stimulus, while the minus lenses increase the accommodative stimulus. The convergence stimulus remains constant, so a change in accommodative convergence must be accompanied by an equal magnitude but opposite direction change in fusional vergence. Therefore, binocular lens rock training may improve fusional vergence as well as accommodative facility.

With a target at 40 cm and +2.00/−2.00D flippers, the accommodative stimulus alternates between 0.50 and 4.50 D, while the total convergence stimulus remains constant at 15Δ. This is illustrated in Figure 14.8.

MONOCULAR LENS ROCK

Because binocular lens rock performance may be limited by fusional vergence, a training program for accommodative facility is sometimes

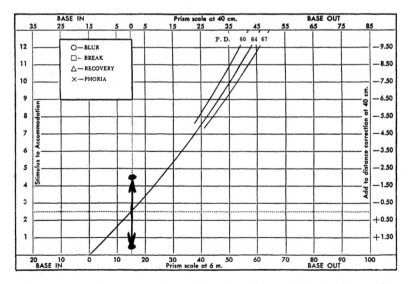

Figure 14.8 Change in accommodative stimulus on binocular lens rock training with a target at 40 cm and +2.00/−2.00D flippers.

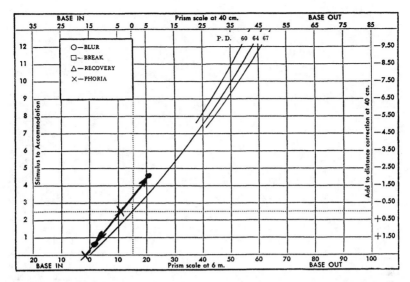

Figure 14.9 Example of the change in accommodative stimulus and convergence position of the eyes on monocular lens rock training with a target at 40 cm and +2.00/−2.00D flippers.

begun with monocular lens rock. This is performed in the same way as binocular lens rock, except that one eye is excluded from viewing by occlusion or some other means.

If a target distance of 40 cm is used with +2.00/−2.00D flippers, the accommodative stimulus changes back and forth between 0.50 and 4.50D. Since binocular fusion is prevented, the convergence position the eyes assume is the phoria position. Therefore, accommodative and convergence stimuli can be represented as moving up and down the phoria line, as shown in Figure 14.9.

DISTANCE ROCK

Accommodative facility training also can be done with a distance rock procedure. The patient alternates fixation between a distance target and a near target. The targets should contain letters or figures close to the patient's best corrected visual acuity. Hart charts (Figure 14.10) are examples of charts often used for this purpose. The patient clears one letter on the distance chart and then clears one letter on the near chart, alternating between them as quickly as possible. With the charts placed at 6 m and 40 cm, the accommodative and convergence stimuli would be at the levels illustrated in Figure 14.11.

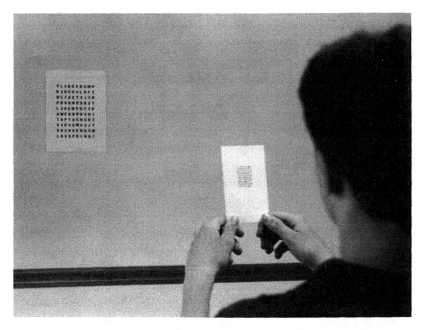

Figure 14.10 Distance rock training with Hart charts.

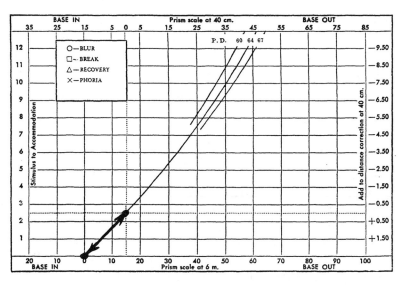

Figure 14.11 Accommodative and convergence stimulus levels for distance rock training with targets at 6 m and 40 cm.

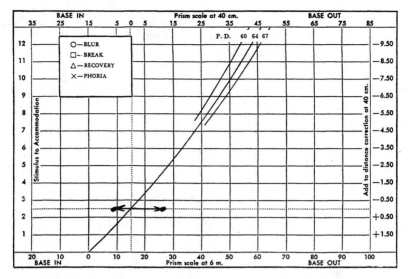

Figure 14.12 Change in convergence stimulus on prism flipper training with a 40-cm target distance and a 6Δ base-in/12Δ base-out flipper.

PRISM ROCK

Vergence facility can be trained by prisms in a flipper bar like that used for lens rock training. The patient is instructed to fuse the two images as quickly as possible after each flip of the flipper. Accommodative stimulus is constant. Base-out prisms on one side of the flipper increase the convergence stimulus for a near target, and the base-in prisms on the other side decrease the convergence stimulus. If a target distance of 40 cm is used with a flipper containing a total of 6Δ base-in on one side and 14Δ base-out on the other, the convergence stimulus would alternate between the levels illustrated in Figure 14.12.

TARGETS FOR CHIASTOPIC FUSION EXERCISES

"Chiastopic fusion" is fusion achieved by converging to fixate two laterally separated targets, similar enough to be fused, such that the right eye fixates the left target and the left eye fixates the right target.[11] Examples of chiastopic fusion targets are displayed in Figure 14.13. Exercises involving chiastopic fusion are used to improve positive fusional convergence. The base-out stimulus on vectograms and tranaglyphs also requires chiastopic fusion. During chiastopic fusion exercises the accommodative stimulus remains constant and depends on the distance from the spectacle plane to the target. The convergence stimulus depends on

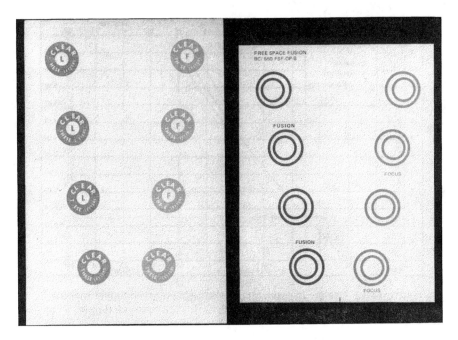

Figure 14.13 Examples of targets used for chiastopic fusion exercises.

the target distance and the amount of lateral separation of the fused targets, a greater lateral separation yielding a greater convergence stimulus.

SPECIFICATION OF A VISION TRAINING PROGRAM BY GRAPHICAL ANALYSIS

Arrows can be used on the graph to specify the type and goal of vision training. The ZCSBV at the beginning of the training program can be plotted. When the numerical goals of the training program have been established, such as by Sheard's criterion in exophoria or by Percival's criterion or the 1:1 rule in esophoria, arrows can be drawn to indicate the improvements desired.

Figure 14.14 presents an example of convergence insufficiency, with arrows describing the fundamentals of the vision training program to be used. Sheard's criterion indicates that the base-out limit at 40 cm should be increased to 24Δ. An arrow at the 2.50D stimulus to accommodation level shows this. The dashed line indicates the goal of the vision training. Its location was suggested by Sheard's criterion applied to the 40-cm findings. It is drawn parallel to the measured base-out limit line (right side of the ZCSBV) since with base-out training the positive width of the ZCSBV is increased. The slope of the line may change slightly if proximal convergence is affected by the training. If the positive width is in-

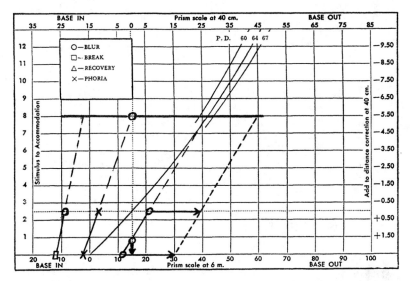

Figure 14.14 An example of how arrows can be used on the graph to describe vision training.

	Phoria	Base-in	Base-out	Plus-to-Blur	Minus-to-Blur
	2 exophoria	X/12/4	12/18/2		
40 cm	12 exophoria	24/38/17	6/12/2	+1.75	−5.50

Amplitude of accommodation = 8.00D.

creased, we can expect the negative relative accommodation to increase, since it will no longer be limited by the available fusional convergence.

REFERENCES

1. Griffin JR. *Binocular Anomalies—Procedures for Vision Therapy.* 2nd ed. New York, NY: Professional Press; 1982:187–418.
2. Rosner J, Rosner J. *Vision Therapy in a Primary-Care Practice.* New York, NY: Professional Press; 1988.
3. Richman JE, Cron MT. *Guide to Vision Therapy.* South Bend, IN: Bernell Corp; 1988.
4. Birnbaum MH. *Optometric Management of Nearpoint Vision Disorders.* Boston, MA: Butterworth-Heinemann; 1993:281–393.
5. Scheiman M, Wick B. *Clinical Management of Binocular Vision-Heterophoric, Accommodative, and Eye Movement Disorders.* Philadelphia, PA: Lippincott; 1994: 107–378.

6. Hofstetter HW. Orthoptics specification by a graphical method. *Am J Optom Arch Am Acad Optom*. 1949;26:439–444.
7. Flom MC. The use of accommodative convergence relationship in prescribing orthoptics. *California Optometrist*. 1953;21:72–75.
8. Schapero M. The characteristics of ten basic visual training problems. *Am J Optom Arch Am Acad Optom*. 1955;32:333–342.
9. Heath GG. The use of graphic analysis in visual training. *Am J Optom Arch Am Acad Optom*. 1959;36:337–350.
10. Borish IM. *Clinical Refraction*. 3rd ed. Boston, MA: Butterworth-Heinemann; 1970:917–923.
11. Cline D, Hofstetter HW, Griffin JR. *Dictionary of Visual Science*. 4th ed. Radnor, PA: Chilton; 1989:285.

SUGGESTED READING

Cooper J. Accommodative dysfunction. In: Amos JF, ed. *Diagnosis and Management in Vision Care*. Boston, MA: Butterworth-Heinemann; 1987:431–459.

Grisham JD. Treatment of binocular dysfunctions. In: Schor CM, Ciuffreda KJ, eds. *Vergence Eye Movements: Basic and Clinical Aspects*. Boston, MA: Butterworth-Heinemann; 1983:605–646.

Hofstetter HW. Orthoptics specification by a graphical method. *Am J Optom Arch Am Acad Optom*. 1949;26:439–444.

Wick BC. Horizontal deviations. In: Amos JF, ed. *Diagnosis and Management in Vision Care*. Boston, MA: Butterworth-Heinemann; 1987:461–510.

PRACTICE PROBLEMS

1. Patient CF

   a. Graph the findings in the following table and indicate by arrows what vision training, as quantified by Sheard's criterion, you would provide.
   b. On the basis of the findings you have available, do you expect this training program to be successful? Why?

	Phoria	Base-in	Base-out	Plus-to-Blur	Minus-to-Blur
6 m	0	X/14/8	18/26/16		
40 cm	10 exophoria	24/28/20	9/16/4	+2.50	−4.50
40 cm +1.00	12 exophoria				

Amplitude of accommodation = 7.00D, PD = 64 mm.

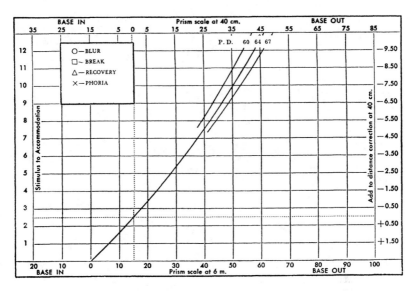

Patient CF

2. Indicate the change in accommodative and convergence stimuli for distance rock accommodative facility training performed monocularly with targets at 6 m and 33 cm for a patient with phorias equal to those in Morgan's norms.

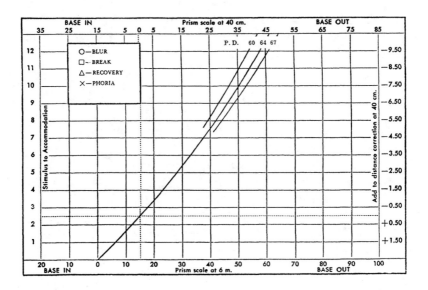

15

Further Consideration of Accommodation, Convergence, and Their Interactions

One of the most interesting and challenging areas of vision science is the study of accommodation and convergence and their interrelationships. So far we have only scratched the surface in our study of clinical graphical analysis. Now we will examine some additional elements of this topic that have clinical import.

FUNCTIONS WITHIN THE ZONE OF CLEAR SINGLE BINOCULAR VISION

It is possible to isolate certain aspects of the relationships between accommodation and convergence by various clinical and experimental techniques. We will look at these functions separately in terms of the stimuli that are used to elicit them.

First, the conditions present during the measurement of clinical base-in and base-out limits are stimulus to accommodation (usually fixation letters), binocular fusion, and convergence movements stimulated by increasing base-in or base-out prism. The patient is asked to report when the letters blur and when they break into two.

The blur indicates that a change in accommodative response has occurred even though there has been no change in the stimulus to accommodation. If the accommodative response versus the convergence demand is plotted for an accommodative stimulus that is neither 0 nor at the individual's maximum level of accommodation, the result is as shown in Figure 15.1. When the plotting is repeated for several different levels of stimulus to accommodation,[1-3] the result is as shown in Figure 15.2.

These figures indicate that the fusional ranges are extended by accommodative convergence. On the base-out side, accommodation increases, causing convergence. On the base-in side, accommodation decreases, causing divergence. Accommodation can change a small amount while retaining clear vision because of depth of focus.

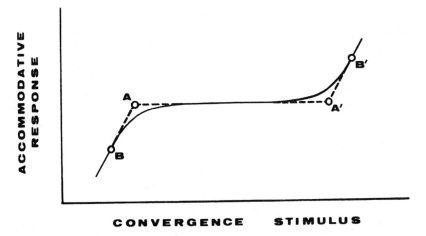

Figure 15.1 The typical change in accommodative response as prism power (convergence stimulus) is varied across the range of single vision with a constant stimulus to accommodation.

(Adapted with permission from Alpern M. Vergence movements. In: Hugh Davson, ed. *Muscular Mechanisms*. Vol 3 of *The Eye*. New York, NY: Academic; 1969:129.)

In Figure 15.1, the B points are the points at which blurs occur; the ends of the curve are where the breaks occur. The vertical distance from one B to the other indicates the individual's depth of focus. In addition, if the ends and the middle portion of the curve are extended, the extensions meet at A. The horizontal distance from A to A' represents the true fusional amplitude; the horizontal distances from A to B represent the extent to which the measured fusional amplitudes are increased by accommodative convergence.

Second, the phoria line is determined by measuring phorias at various levels of accommodation. The conditions present during phoria testing are absence of binocular fusion and a stimulus to accommodation. The reciprocal of the slope of the phoria line is the ACA ratio; that is, the slope of the phoria line is determined by accommodative convergence.

In Figure 15.2 the phoria line is linear, except for the portion close to the top of the zone of clear single binocular vision (ZCSBV), or, in other words, at levels of accommodation close to the amplitude of accommodation.[4] It has been suggested that the little curved portion at the top occurs because more innervation to accommodation is required for the maximum levels of accommodation response and, as a result, the innervation to accommodative convergence is greater at that level. There also may be some nonlinearity at low levels (0–1.00D) of accommodative stimulus. Over intermediate levels, there is a high degree of linearity.[5]

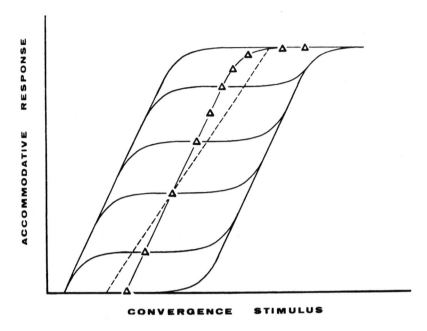

Figure 15.2 The ZCSBV plotted as accommodative response versus convergence stimulus for various constant levels of stimulus to accommodation. The dashed line is the demand line. The phoria line connects the Δs, which are single phoria measurements. By estimation from the graph, this individual appears to have an ACA ratio between 4 and 5Δ/D.

(Adapted with permission from Alpern M. Vergence movements. In Hugh Davson, ed. *Muscular Mechanisms*. Vol 3 of *The Eye*. New York, NY: Academic; 1969:159.)

A third function that can be plotted within the ZCSBV is convergence accommodation,[6] which is the accommodation induced by or associated with convergence. The required conditions are binocular fusion, absence of a stimulus to accommodation, and stimulation of convergence by increasing base-in prism followed by base-out prism. Curves for convergence accommodation are presented in Figure 15.3, which also illustrates that the slope of the convergence accommodation curve changes in presbyopia, whereas the slope of the phoria line does not.[5]

The slope of the convergence accommodation line has been called the CAC ratio. The CAC ratio is the ratio of change in convergence accommodation (CA) to change in convergence (C). The CAC ratio is not usually determined clinically, but it could be measured by doing the binocular cross-cylinder test through different amounts of prism or by performing Nott or monocular estimation method dynamic retinoscopy at different prism settings while the patient views a target that does not contain an adequate stimulus for the control of optical reflex accommodation.[7–10]

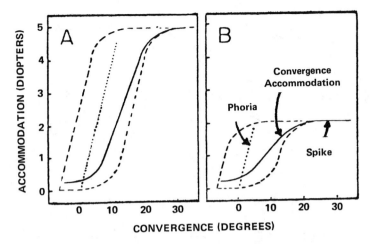

Figure 15.3 The ZCSBV with phoria line and convergence accommodation curve plotted inside. The diagram indicates how the change in slope of the convergence accommodation is associated with aging while the slope of the phoria line remains constant.

(Reprinted with permission from Balsam MD, Fry GA. Convergence accommodation. *Am J Optom Arch Am Acad Optom.* 1959;36:567–575.)

An example of a clinically derived CAC ratio is given in Figure 15.4. With a 6Δ base-in prism in place, the binocular cross-cylinder end-point is +1.00D over the subjective refraction to best visual acuity. The convergence stimulus for this point is 15Δ − 6Δ = 9Δ. The accommodative stimulus is 2.50D −1.00D = 1.50D. This and the other two points are plotted on the graph in Figure 15.4. Accommodation changed 0.25D for each 6Δ change in convergence. Therefore, the slope of the line, the CAC ratio, is 0.06 D/Δ.

Daum et al[9] reported a mean CAC ratio of 0.06 D/Δ. The mean slope of the convergence accommodation line (CAC ratio) is less than the mean slope of the phoria line (inverse of the ACA ratio).[9,10]

Theories of Disparity-Induced Accommodation (Convergence Accommodation)

Because the physiologic basis of convergence accommodation is not known for certain, it is sometimes referred to as "disparity-induced accommodation."[11] Such terminology implies that retinal disparity can induce a change in accommodation, whereas the use of the term "convergence accommodation" seems to imply that it is the process of convergence that causes a change in accommodation.

The fact that the phoria line and the convergence accommodation curve do not coincide may suggest that accommodative convergence and convergence accommodation are separate neurologic entities. However,

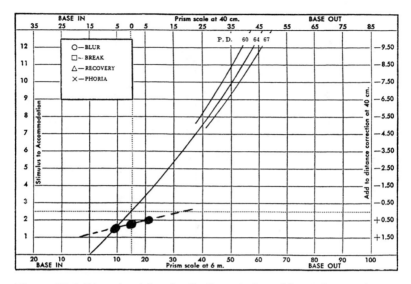

Figure 15.4 Example of the plot findings (indicated by circles) used in the determination of a clinically derived CAC ratio. The following test results were obtained using a 40-cm target distance.

Prism Setting	Binocular Cross-Cylinder Test Results (plus over the subjective refraction to best visual acuity)
6Δ base-in	+1.00D
0	+0.75D
6Δ base-out	+0.50D

PD = 64 mm.

it also may be possible that the convergence occurring during the elicitation of the convergence accommodation curve is simply a combination of accommodative convergence and fusional convergence. Since there is no stimulus to accommodation present, accommodative convergence can be used along with fusional convergence without inducing a blur. To clarify this concept, Fry[3] called accommodative convergence "triad convergence" to indicate that accommodation, convergence, and pupil constriction occur together. Convergence accommodation, then, is the accommodation that occurs with triad convergence, and the convergence occurring under these conditions is a combination of triad convergence and fusional convergence, no accommodation being associated with fusional convergence.

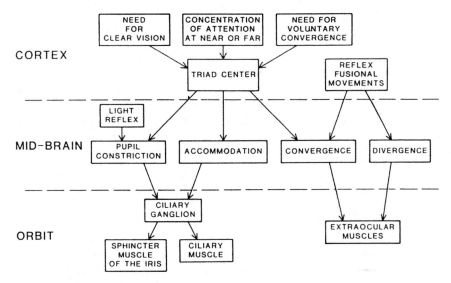

Figure 15.5 A diagram illustrating the neural mechanisms proposed by Fry for accommodation and convergence.

(Reprinted with permission from Fry GA. Basic concepts underlying graphical analysis. In: Schor CM, Ciuffreda KJ, eds. *Vergence Eye Movements: Basic and Clinical Aspects.* Boston, MA: Butterworth-Heinemann; 1983:403–437.)

A diagram illustrating Fry's concept is given in Figure 15.5.

Another theory is that accommodative convergence and convergence accommodation are separate neural elements.[12-15] A change in accommodation induces a change in accommodative convergence, and a change in convergence in response to retinal disparity induces a change in convergence accommodation. A diagram proposed by Schor to illustrate the dual interaction of accommodation and convergence is shown in Figure 15.6.

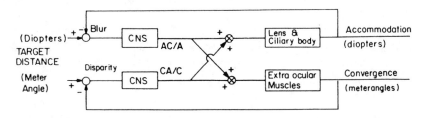

Figure 15.6 A diagram illustrating the mechanisms for interaction of accommodation and convergence proposed by Schor.

(Reprinted with permission from Schor CM. Models of mutual interaction between accommodation and convergence. *Am J Optom Physiol Opt.* 1985;62:369–374.)

DEPTH OF FOCUS EFFECTS ON THE ZONE OF CLEAR SINGLE BINOCULAR VISION

Depth of focus makes clear vision possible even when there is a (small) lag or lead of accommodation. We have already seen that during a fusional vergence amplitude measurement accommodative convergence is used in addition to fusional convergence. A blur occurs when accommodation has shifted the depth of field such that the object of regard is no longer within it. As we can visualize from Figure 15.2, if we plotted a ZCSBV with accommodative response values rather than stimulus values, the base-out blur points would be shifted up by an amount limited by the depth of focus, because accommodative convergence is being used. Likewise, the base-in blur points would be shifted down because accommodative divergence is being brought into play.

At other than 0 stimulus to accommodation levels, accommodative divergence can supplement negative fusional convergence. At 0 stimulus to accommodation, accommodative divergence cannot be used because, presumably, accommodation is already relaxed. This situation has two effects on the ZCSBV. First, it explains why a break without a blur can be expected on the base-in fusional amplitude measurement at distance. If a blur is obtained on this test, the patient may have been underplussed or over-minused on the refraction. Second, the situation may make the ZCSBV narrower at the 0 stimulus to accommodation level than at other accommodation levels. Thus, depth of focus can contribute to a fanning-out of the ZCSBV, just as proximal convergence (discussed in Chapter 4) does.

Tests of accommodation (negative relative accommodation, positive relative accommodation, and amplitude) also are influenced by the depth of focus. For a person with a large depth of focus (such as from a small pupil diameter), the negative relative accommodation may extend below the bottom of the graph. For a patient with a moderate to large pupil diameter, if the negative relative accommodation point extends substantially below the 0 stimulus to accommodation line (negative relative accommodation at 40 cm greater than approximately 3.00D), the suspicion is of too much minus or not enough plus on the refraction. Depth of focus also explains why a greater than 0 amplitude of accommodation is obtained for an absolute presbyope.

PRISM ADAPTATION

The phenomenon responsible for a shift in phorias after binocular viewing through prisms is prism adaptation. Base-in prism causes an exo shift and base-out prism causes an eso shift. Theories of its physiologic basis include after-discharge of innervation to the extraocular muscles[2] and motor adaptation of tonic convergence.[16] Since prism adaptation is elicited by the use of fusional convergence, Alpern[2] called it "fusional aftereffect" and Schor[14] called it "slow fusional vergence." It also has been called "vergence adaptation." In terms of its effects on the ZCSBV, perhaps it is best to think of prism adaptation as an adjustment in the level of tonic convergence and, thus, lateral position of the zone.

In most individuals, adaptation to base-out prism is greater than adaptation to base-in prism. For this reason, some optometrists recommend taking base-in fusional vergence amplitudes before base-out. All optometrists agree that phorias should be measured before fusional amplitudes so that the effect of prism adaptation on the phorias will be minimized.

There are considerable differences in the extent to which prism adaptation is present in different individuals. It is a useful adaptation in that persons who exhibit a great deal of it are generally asymptomatic.

STABILITY OF THE ACA RATIO AND THE COMPONENTS OF CONVERGENCE

There is some confusion about how alterable phorias and ACA ratios are. This situation is largely due to terminology problems and misinterpretations of study results. Perhaps the best way to view this question is in terms of the Maddox components of convergence. Prism adaptation can be thought of as an adaptation of tonic convergence.[16] Proximal convergence, in terms of a PCT ratio (proximal convergence to test distance ratio, expressed in prism diopters per diopter), is quite often changed by orthoptics.[17,18] The amount of accommodative convergence in play during a phoria measurement is a function of the accommodative response as predicted by the ACA ratio. Thus, a phoria can be changed by prism adaptation, proximal convergence, or changes in the lag of accommodation. In the absence of changes in these factors, the phoria is quite stable. The fourth of the Maddox components of convergence (fusional convergence) is, of course, readily changed by orthoptics.

Most of the confusion about the stability of the ACA ratio and its amenability to change through orthoptics has resulted from not distinguishing between stimulus and response ACA ratios. Most studies of response ACA ratios have shown stability over time and minimal change with orthoptics, whereas many studies with stimulus ACA ratios have had different results.[5] Thus, variation in a given patient's clinically measured ACA is more likely to be due to changes in lag of accommodation than to changes in the neural interaction of accommodation and convergence. If distance and near phorias are used, changes in proximal convergence also may cause apparent instability of the ACA.

In one study,[19] a small change in response ACA ratio (mean, $0.66\Delta D$) was demonstrated in eight subjects during an orthoptics program. One year following the cessation of the orthoptics program, the ACA ratios had returned to the levels measured at the beginning of the training.

DRUG EFFECTS ON THE ACA RATIO

Some drugs will temporarily change the ACA ratio by their effects on accommodation or on the central nervous system. Most of what we know about the effects of autonomic agents applied topically to the eye come from their use in accommodative esotropia, which is characterized by moderate to high hyperopia and a high ACA ratio. The typical accommodative esotrope can be viewed as a convergence excess patient whose hyperopia results in strabismus when it is uncorrected.

Parasympathomimetic drugs allow a given level of innervation to the ciliary muscle to yield a greater dioptric amount of accommodation. Since topically applied parasympathomimetics have their effects on the ciliary muscle but not on the extraocular muscles, stimulation of the near triad causes relatively easier accommodation than before drug application; accommodative convergence is unaffected. Thus, the ACA ratio is reduced as long as the drug is active.

Parasympatholytic drugs have a cycloplegic effect; that is, they paralyze the ciliary muscle. When innervation to accommodation and accommodative convergence occurs after application of a parasympatholytic drug, accommodative convergence proceeds as usual, but accommodation is paralyzed. As a result, the ACA ratio increases dramatically. The time course of the ACA ratio change is directly related to the time course of the cycloplegic effect of the drugs.[2]

Parasympathomimetics are used in accommodative esotropia because they temporarily reduce the ACA ratio.[4] Parasympatholytics are used in accommodative esotropia because the patient learns to stop trying to accommodate; in a patient who does try to accommodate, the esotropia becomes worse because the ACA ratio is higher.[4] A more common management of accommodative esotropia is full plus at distance, a plus add, orthoptics, and perhaps base-out prism.

A drug with well-known central nervous system effects on the ACA ratio is ethyl alcohol,[20] which causes a dose-related reduction in the ACA ratio as well as an increase in tonic convergence and a reduction in fusional vergence amplitudes. As the level of intoxication increases, the ability to retain single vision decreases, because distance esophoria increases, near-point exophoria increases, and fusional reserves decrease.

PROXIMAL ACCOMMODATION AND
PROXIMAL CONVERGENCE

The change in convergence associated with a change in viewing distance is composed of changes in accommodative convergence, proximal convergence, and fusional convergence. Each of these components is important in the total vergence response.[21] Likewise, accommodation responds to proximity cues or awareness of nearness in addition to optical defocus. The former is often called "proximal accommodation," and the latter is referred to as "optical reflex accommodation."

Because proximity cues are important in accommodation and convergence responses, many clinicians will emphasize the awareness of changes of perceived distance and size during vision training programs. For instance, the SILO response will be brought to the patient's attention. The SILO response is the appearance of a target getting smaller and closer associated with convergence occurring in response to increasing base-out prism, and the appearance of a target getting larger and farther away during divergence stimulated by increasing base-in prism. The amount of proximal convergence occurring with a given change in test distance can be changed with vision training.[17]

The ratio of change in proximal convergence to change in test distance is often referred to as the PCT ratio,[18] which is measured in prism diopters per diopter. One method that has been used to derive PCT ratios is to subtract the gradient ACA ratio (which does not include changes in distance) from the calculated ACA ratio (which does involve changes in distance). If we use Morgan's norms for the determination of a PCT ratio, one finds

$$\text{PCT ratio} = \text{calculated ACA} - \text{gradient ACA}$$
$$= 5.2\Delta/\text{D} - 4\Delta/\text{D}$$
$$= 1.2\Delta/\text{D}$$

Mean PCT ratios reported in the literature have varied from 0.7 to $2\Delta/\text{D}$,[18] with ratios derived binocularly often being greater than ratios derived monocularly.[22]

Rosenfield et al[23] reported that proximal accommodation and proximal convergence are constant at a minimum for targets at or beyond 3 m. They also reported that both proximal accommodation and proximal convergence change linearly with target distance expressed in diopters or meter angles for objects closer than 3 m. (The meter angle is an angular unit for convergence in which one meter angle is a reciprocal meter. It is usually measured from the spectacle plane. Diopters and meter angles are thus equal in magnitude for a given target distance.)

DARK FOCUS AND DARK VERGENCE

When sufficient cues for optical reflex accommodation are not present, such as in darkness or in empty visual field, accommodation focuses for an intermediate distance. The amount of accommodation occurring in darkness is known as the "dark focus." Leibowitz and Owens[24] found a mean dark focus of 1.52D (SD = 0.77D) in 220 college students. This accommodation in darkness is responsible for the phenomenon known as "night myopia."[25–27]

A potential clinical method for measuring the dark focus is performing retinoscopy in a darkened room. Results from retinoscopy done in a dark room have been reported to correlate with laboratory measurements of dark focus.[28,29] Clinical determination of dark focus may aid in prescribing lenses for patients bothered by night myopia, such as when driving at night.[27,30]

The vergence position of the eyes in darkness also has been studied; this often is referred to as "dark vergence." The dark vergence position can be predicted by adding the amount of accommodative convergence expected to occur with the dark focus (determined by multiplying the dioptric dark focus by the ACA ratio) to the distance phoria.[31,32] As we have discussed, the distance phoria is the physiologic position of rest of the eyes when accommodation is at a zero level. Thus, we can say that the dark vergence is determined by the physiologic position of rest and the accommodative convergence that is associated with the accommodation that occurs in the dark.

The dark focus level for a given individual is relatively stable over time.[33,34] However, dark focus increases after near fixation for a few minutes or more and dark focus decreases after distance fixation.[35–38] Some investigators think of this shift in dark focus in the direction of the fixation distance as an accommodative adaptation, analogous in function to prism adaptation in the vergence system.

Accommodation is controlled by the opposing actions of the parasympathetic and sympathetic divisions of the autonomic nervous system.[39,40] Experimentation and a review of the literature led Gilmartin and Hogan[41,42] to conclude that variability in dark focus is due to variability in parasympathetic rather than sympathetic ciliary muscle tone.

VERGENCE FACILITY

Vergence facility was mentioned earlier in Chapters 11 and 14. Although it is not a standard clinical test, some clinicians recommend its use. Grisham[43] found that fusional vergence latencies were greater and fusional vergence velocities were less in subjects who had abnormal vergence and phoria findings based on Morgan's norms compared with subjects who had normal findings.

Grisham[44] recommends a test in which the clinician observes the latency and velocity of a fusional vergence eye movement. A 6Δ base-out prism is introduced in front of one eye while the patient views a target at approximately 40 cm. The clinician carefully watches the eye without the prism, and subjectively evaluates the latency and velocity of the fusional vergence response. Grisham emphasizes that experience with the technique is necessary to discern whether the response is slow, moderate, or fast.

Vergence facility testing also has been done with prism flippers. Buzzelli[45] tested 310 schoolchildren using 4Δ base-in/16Δ base-out flippers while they viewed an anaglyph target at 40 cm. Test performance improved with age. For example, 5-year-olds had a mean of 7.6 cycles per minute (SD = 1.2) and 12-year-olds had a mean of 13.0 cycles per minute (SD = 1.2). Delgadillo and Griffin[46] tested 26 nonpresbyopic optometry students with 8Δ base-in/8Δ base-out and 5Δ base-in/15Δ base-out flippers using a vectographic target at 40 cm. Mean values were presented for both tests and for different testing sequences. The mean values were similar for the two tests, ranging from 11.3 to 14.1 cycles per minute (SD = 4.0 to 5.7). Further studies for standardization of vergence facility testing would be helpful.

GETTING TO KNOW THE GRAPH BETTER

Now that you are accomplished plotters of optometric findings, it might be useful to review the first few chapters to better understand the construction of graphs, the scales on the graphs, the basis for the plotting of various findings, and so on. As indicated earlier, the scale at the bottom of the graph is an absolute scale, with 0 indicating parallelism of the lines of sight, values to the left of 0 indicating divergence from parallelism, and values to the right of 0 indicating various levels of convergence of the lines of sight. From this, we can think of the positions of the lines of sight as being in space rather than as being merely points marked on a paper. We can determine how much the eyes converge or diverge during any given test. For example, if an individual with a 64-mm PD measures 8Δ exophoria at 40 cm, the eyes are actually converged 7Δ during that test: 15 + (−8) = 7.

One of the uses of graphical analysis discussed in Chapter 1 is the prediction of test results. The demand line represents the stimulus to accommodation and the convergence stimulus for objects at various distances when the patient is looking through lenses equal in power to the subjective refraction. When lens power is varied from the subjective refraction, the stimulus to accommodation changes but the convergence stimulus remains the same for a given distance. Thus, to predict performance through various adds, one simply moves straight up (for minus spherical lens changes) or straight down (for plus) from the demand line point for the test distance in question and observes the relationship of the ZCSBV to this point. This procedure can be used to confirm observations about the patient's status without the spherical correction as well as to help in deciding whether to use an add or an alteration in lens power in the spectacle lenses prescribed.

Chapter 3 discussed the five geometric properties of the ZCSBV and their clinical correlates. The slope of the ZCSBV is correlated with the inverse of the ACA ratio. The ACA ratio represents the amount of accommodative convergence (AC) occurring with a given amount of accommodation (A). Convergence is given on the x-axis and accommodation on the y-axis, so the ACA ratio can be calculated as $\Delta x/\Delta y$. This is what is done in many laboratory studies of response ACAs: several phorias are plotted at intermediate accommodative stimulus levels, and the slope of the phoria line is calculated with such statistical methods as linear regression analysis. Clinically, we can easily do much the same thing. If several phorias are plotted, we can draw a best-fitting straight line through them by visual inspection and calculate the inverse of the slope using the scale values on the graph. In addition, any two phorias, regardless of the lens powers or distances used, can be employed to calculate ACA ratios:

$$\text{ACA ratio} = \frac{\begin{array}{c}(\text{convergence stimulus \#1} + \text{phoria \#1}) - \\ (\text{convergence stimulus \#2} + \text{phoria \#2})\end{array}}{\begin{array}{c}\text{stimulus to accommodation \#1} - \\ \text{stimulus to accommodation \#2}\end{array}}$$

The formulas for calculated and gradient ACA ratios are simplifications of this formula. The ACA relationship is highly linear, but some nonlinearity may appear in clinically derived phoria lines as a result of poorly controlled accommodation on some phorias or proximal convergence when both test distance and lens power are varied.

ALTERNATIVE FORMS OF THE GRAPH

The clinical graph for accommodation and convergence data has been presented in different forms on occasion. One variation is the use of the spectacle plane rather than the ocular centers of rotation for computation of convergence values. The demand line then becomes linear. Sometimes different units have been used for convergence, as for example, degrees, centrads, or meter angles.[47] If meter angles are used, the demand line becomes a 1:1 line, the number of meter angles of convergence stimulus equaling the number of diopters of accommodative stimulus for each fixation distance. Sometimes accommodation is represented on the x-axis and convergence on the y-axis.[10,48]

A NOTE ON ASTHENOPIA

In investigating the potential sources of asthenopia, we can say that of the Maddox components of convergence, asthenopia is related to stress on fusional convergence.[33] The usefulness of clinical guidelines such as Sheard's criterion or of fixation disparity data is attributable to the fact that they are related to the stress on fusional convergence. Because poor accommodation skills can cause ocular discomfort, the clinician should examine all areas of accommodative function in patients with asthenopia.

Asthenopia also can result from uncorrected refractive conditions, such as hyperopia, astigmatism, and anisometropia and, in some cases, from the consequences of correcting a refractive error, such as in correction-induced aniseikonia. Birnbaum[49,50] also has proposed a physiologic mechanism by which stress and psychological factors may play a role in producing asthenopia.

GRAPHICAL ANALYSIS IN STRABISMUS

Clinical findings also can be portrayed graphically in strabismic cases. This portrayal can be of use in determining the prognosis and designing a program of orthoptics. A strabismus is noted whenever the demand line falls outside the ZCSBV, that is, anytime it falls outside the break lines. In everyday vision it is probably more realistic to say that the strabismus exists at all distances at which the demand line does not lie within the lateral limits of the ZCSBV. In the artificial conditions of the phoropter, most patients will give up clear vision to retain single vision (and thus will report a blur before a break).

An example of strabismus findings is given in Figure 15.7. The symbols used in this figure are the same as those used previously. The magnitude of a tropia is marked with an X, as is the magnitude of a phoria. The line through these points is called the "phoria-tropia line" when both phorias and tropias are represented or the "tropia line" when only

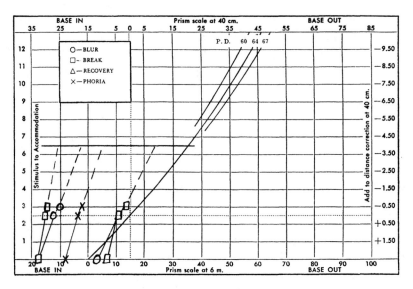

Figure 15.7 An example of graphical analysis in strabismus.

	Phoria/Tropia	Base-in	Base-out
6 m	8 exophoria	X/18/10	2/6/−2
40 cm	17 exotropia	26/30/20	X/−4/−10
33 cm	20 exotropia	28/34/20	x/−6/−10

Amplitude of accommodation = 6.50D.

tropias are represented. In Figure 15.7 an exophoria is noted at distance, whereas an exotropia is noted at 40 cm and at 33 cm. To determine the distance within which a strabismus is manifest, one can find the point at which the demand line crosses outside the blur or blur-break line. In this example, the point is approximately at the 1.25D stimulus to accommodation level. Converting this to a distance one gets approximately 80 cm. Therefore, graphical analysis suggests that this individual has a tropia anywhere within about 80 cm from the eyes.

Strabismus often is more than just a motor phenomenon. Frequently, there are attendant sensory anomalies. One of these anomalies is suppression. If the suppression is deep, the patient may have a total lack of sensory fusion, which results in an absence of fusional amplitude (motor fusion). The effect on graphical analysis is that such an individual does not have a ZCSBV. However, the tropia line can still be plotted and an ACA ratio can still be calculated. In fact, determination of the ACA ratio is an essential part of strabismus diagnosis. The ACA ratio and the graph can be used to predict the amount of minus add (exotropes) or plus add (esotropes) that will produce lateral orthotropia at a given distance.

Another sensory anomaly that may accompany strabismus is anomalous retinal correspondence, which is present when the amount of tropia measured objectively (objective angle of strabismus) differs significantly from the amount of tropia measured subjectively (subjective angle of strabismus). The difference between the objective angle and the subjective angle is the angle of anomaly. In anomalous retinal correspondence, both an objective tropia line and a subjective tropia line could be plotted. The distance between them on the graph represents the angle of anomaly. In the normal condition, called normal retinal correspondence, the subjective angle is equal to the objective angle within the limits of clinical measurement errors.

REFERENCES

1. Fry GA. Further experiments on the accommodation- convergence relationship. *Am J Optom Arch Am Acad Optom.* 1939;16:325–336.
2. Alpern M. Types of movement. In: Davson H, ed. *Muscular Mechanisms.* 2nd ed. Vol 3 of *The Eye.* New York, NY: Academic; 1969:65–174.
3. Fry GA. Basic concepts underlying graphical analysis. In: Schor CM, Ciuffreda KJ, eds. *Vergence Eye Movements: Basic and Clinical Aspects.* Boston, MA: Butterworth-Heinemann; 1983:403– 437.
4. Alpern M. The zone of clear single binocular vision at the upper levels of accommodation and convergence. *Am J Optom Arch Am Acad Optom.* 1950;27: 491–513.
5. Ciuffreda KJ, Kenyon RV. Accommodative vergence and accommodation in normals, amblyopes, and strabismics. In: Schor CM, Ciuffreda KJ, eds. *Vergence Eye Movements: Basic and Clinical Aspects.* Boston, MA: Butterworth-Heinemann; 1983:101–173.
6. Balsam MD, Fry GA. Convergence accommodation. *Am J Optom Arch Am Acad Optom.* 1959;36:567–575.
7. Schor CM, Narayan V. Graphical analysis of prism adaptation, convergence accommodation, and accommodative convergence. *Am J Optom Physiol Opt.* 1982;59:774–784.
8. Tsuetaki TX, Schor CM. Clinical method for measuring adaptation of tonic accommodation and vergence accommodation. *Am J Optom Physiol Opt.* 1987; 64:437–449.
9. Daum KM, Rutstein RP, Houston G IV, Clore HA, Corliss DA. Evaluation of a new criterion of binocularity. *Optom Vis Sci.* 1989;66:218–228.
10. Goss DA. Pratt system of clinical analysis of accommodation and convergence. *Optom Vis Sci.* 1989;66:805–806.

11. Rosenfield M, Gilmartin B. Disparity-induced accommodation in late-onset myopia. *Ophthal Physiol Opt.* 1988;8:353–355.

12. Semmlow IL. Oculomotor responses to near stimuli: the near triad. In: Zuber BL, ed. *Models of Oculomotor Behavior and Control.* Boca Raton, FL: CRC Press; 1981:161–191.

13. Semmlow JL, Hung GK. The near response: theories of control. In: Schor CM, Ciuffreda KJ, eds. *Vergence Eye Movements: Basic and Clinical Aspects.* Boston, MA: Butterworth-Heinemann; 1983:175–195.

14. Schor CM. Fixation disparity and vergence adaptation. In: Schor CM, Ciuffreda KJ, eds. *Vergence Eye: Basic and Clinical Aspects.* Boston, MA: Butterworth-Heinemann; 1983:465–516.

15. Schor CM. Models of mutual interaction between accommodation and convergence. *Am J Optom Physiol Opt.* 1985;62:369–374.

16. Owens DA, Leibowitz HW. Perceptual and motor consequences of tonic vergence. In: Schor CM, Ciuffreda KJ, eds. *Vergence Eye Movements: Basic and Clinical Aspects.* Boston, MA: Butterworth- Heinemann; 1983:25–74.

17. Mannen DL, Bannon MJ, Septon RD. Effects of base-out training on proximal convergence. *Am J Optom Physiol Opt.* 1981;58:1187– 1193.

18. Hokoda SC, Ciuffreda KJ. Theoretical and clinical importance of proximal vergence and accommodation. In: Schor CM, Ciuffreda KJ, eds. *Vergence Eye Movements: Basic and Clinical Aspects.* Boston, MA: Butterworth-Heinemann; 1983: 75–97.

19. Flom MC. On the relationship between accommodation and accommodative convergence: part 3. Effects of orthoptics. *Am J Optom Arch Am Acad Optom.* 1960;37:619–632.

20. Hogan RE, Linfield PB. The effects of moderate doses of ethanol on heterophoria and other aspects of binocular vision. *Ophthal Physiol Opt.* 1983;3: 21–31.

21. North RV, Henson DB, Smith TJ. Influence of proximal, accommodative and disparity stimuli upon the vergence system. *Ophthal Physiol Opt.* 1993;13: 239–243.

22. Joubert C, Bedell HE. Proximal vergence and perceived distance. *Optom Vis Sci.* 1990;67:29–35.

23. Rosenfield M, Ciuffreda KJ, Hung GK. The linearity of proximally induced accommodation and vergence. *Invest Ophthalmol Vis Sci.* 1991;32: 2985–2991.

24. Leibowitz HW, Owens DA. New evidence for the intermediate position of relaxed accommodation. *Doc Ophthalmol.* 1978;46:133– 147.

25. Leibowitz HW, Owens DA. Night myopia and the intermediate dark focus of accommodation. *J Opt Soc Am.* 1975;65:1121–1128.

26. Hope GM, Rubin ML. Night myopia. *Surv Ophthalmol.* 1984;29:129–136.

27. Goss DA, Eskridge JB. Myopia. In: Amos JF, ed. *Diagnosis and Management in Vision Care.* Boston, MA: Butterworth-Heinemann; 1987:121–171.

28. Owens DA, Mohindra I, Held R. Near retinoscopy and the effectiveness of a retinoscope beam as an accommodative stimulus. *Invest Ophthalmol Vis Sci.* 1980;18:942–949.

29. Bullimore MA, Gilmartin B, Hogan RE. Objective and subjective measurement of tonic accommodation. *Ophthal Physiol Opt.* 1986;6:57–62.

30. Owens DA, Leibowitz HW. Night myopia: cause and a possible basis for amelioration. *Am J Optom Physiol Opt.* 1976;53:709–717.

31. Wolf KS, Bedell HE, Pedersen SB. Relations between accommodation and vergence in darkness. *Optom Vis Sci.* 1990;67:89–93.
32. Rosenfield M, Ciuffreda KJ. Distance heterophoria and tonic vergence. *Optom Vis Sci.* 1990;67:667–669.
33. Miller RJ. Temporal stability of the dark focus of accommodation. *Am J Optom Physiol Opt.* 1978;55:447–450.
34. Owens RL, Higgins KE. Long-term stability of the dark focus of accommodation. *Am J Optom Physiol Opt.* 1983;60:32–38.
35. Ebenholtz SM. Accommodative hysteresis: relation to resting focus. *Am J Optom Physiol Opt.* 1985;62:755–762.
36. Ebenholtz SM. Long-term endurance of adaptive shifts in tonic accommodation. *Ophthal Physiol Opt.* 1988;8:427–431.
37. McBrien NA, Millodot M. Differences in adaptation of tonic accommodation with refractive state. *Invest Ophthalmol Vis Sci.* 1988;29:460–469.
38. Gilmartin B, Bullimore M. Adaptation of tonic accommodation to sustained visual tasks in emmetropia and late-onset myopia. *Optom Vis Sci.* 1991;68: 22–26.
39. Cogan DC. Accommodation and the autonomic nervous system. *Arch Ophthalmol.* 1937;18:739–766.
40. Stephens KG. Effect of the sympathetic nervous system on accommodation. *Am J Optom Physiol Opt.* 1985;62:402–406.
41. Gilmartin B, Hogan RE. The relationship between tonic accommodation and ciliary muscle innervation. *Invest Ophthalmol Vis Sci.* 1985;26:1024–1028.
42. Gilmartin B. A review of the role of sympathetic innervation of the ciliary muscle in ocular accommodation. *Ophthal Physiol Opt.* 1986;6:23–37.
43. Grisham JD. The dynamics of fusional vergence eye movements in binocular dysfunction. *Am J Optom Physiol Opt.* 1980;57:645–655.
44. Grisham JD. Treatment of binocular dysfunctions. In: Schor CM, Ciuffreda KJ, eds. *Vergence Eye Movements: Basic and Clinical Aspects.* Boston, MA: Butterworth-Heinemann; 1983:605–646.
45. Buzzelli AR. Vergence facility: developmental trends in a school age population. *Am J Optom Physiol Opt.* 1986;63:351–355.
46. Delgadillo HM, Griffin JR. Vergence facility and associated symptoms: a comparison of two prism flipper tests. *J Behav Optom.* 1992;3:91–94.
47. Hofstetter HW. Graphical analysis. In: Schor CM, Ciuffreda KJ, eds. *Vergence Eye Movements: Basic and Clinical Aspects.* Boston, MA: Butterworth-Heinemann; 1983:439–464.
48. Hofstetter HW. A revised schematic for the graphic analysis of the accommodation-convergence relationship. *Can J Optom.* 1968;30:49–52.
49. Birnbaum MH. Nearpoint visual stress: a physiological model. *J Am Optom Assoc.* 1984;55:825–835.
50. Birnbaum MH. Nearpoint visual stress: clinical implications. *J Am Optom Assoc.* 1985;56:480–490.

SUGGESTED READING

Schor CM, Ciuffreda KJ, eds. *Vergence Eye Movements: Basic and Clinical Aspects.* Boston, MA: Butterworth-Heinemann; 1983.

PRACTICE PROBLEMS

1. Why are phoria measurements typically taken before fusional vergence amplitudes?

2. Which of the Maddox components of convergence can be altered by training?

3. Explain why the fusional vergence amplitudes measured to the blur point include both fusional and accommodative convergence. How does the depth of focus relate to this?

4. What does the demand line represent?

5. Why do cycloplegic drugs affect the ACA ratio? Is their effect permanent?

6. What is the clinical significance of prism adaptation?

7. Patient BL, a strabismic with normal retinal correspondence, but no fusional ranges:

   Tropia at 6 m: 10 exotropia
   Tropia at 40 cm: 16 exotropia

   a. Plot the tropias.
   b. What is the ACA ratio?
   c. At what distances is this patient strabismic?

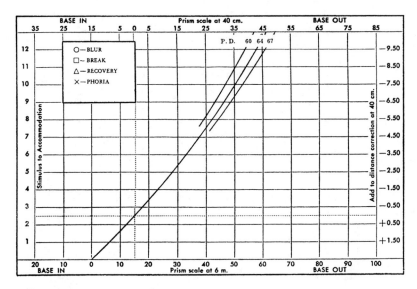

Patient BL

8. Patient DM

    a. With the subjective in place, at what distances does patient DM manifest a strabismus?

    b. Without any lenses, at what distances does the patient probably manifest a strabismus?

    c. What is the ACA ratio?

    d. What lens, prism, or orthoptic therapy would you provide in this case?

    e. Graph this case and indicate on the graph what vision training you would provide.

	Phoria	Base-in	Base-out	Plus-to-Blur	Minus-to-Blur
6 m	7 esophoria	X/4/0	X/26/18		
40 cm	17 esophoria	X/−2/−8	32/38/27		
40 cm + 1.00	7 esophoria	X/6/0	24/32/20	+1.50	−0.75

Amplitude of accommodation = 5.75D. Subjective refraction OD + 1.75 sph; OS + 2.00 − 0.25 − 90; PD = 63 mm.

The tests are done with the subjective refraction in place or the +1.00 add over the subjective, as noted.

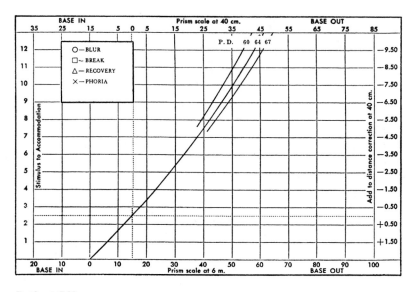

Patient DM

16

Other Systems of Case Analysis

It is important to have a systemic approach to the analysis and diagnosis of accommodation and vergence disorders. One such approach was summarized in Chapters 11 and 13. The analysis of vergence disorders included comparison of findings to norms, identifying a case type, application of the appropriate rules of thumb, and determination of lens, prism, or vision training prescription based on phoria, vergence range, and/or fixation disparity data (see Chapter 11). A systematic analysis of accommodative disorders involves testing all aspects of accommodative function (see Chapter 13). The literature supporting the scientific background and clinical effectiveness of such an approach has been cited in previous chapters. Approaches consistent in many aspects with this one have been described by other clinicians.[1-7]

Many rules of thumb and systems of analysis proposed throughout the years have not been covered in this text. Some of these have been discussed by Borish[8]; a few of them will be described below.

OPTOMETRIC EXTENSION PROGRAM ANALYSIS

The Optometric Extension Program (OEP) is an organization that was formed in the 1920s. Its analysis system was developed by Skeffington and colleagues.[9] The developers and followers of OEP analysis have made some philosophical assumptions concerning accommodation and convergence disorders.[10-12] One of these is that anomalous clinical findings are the result of near-point stress. Prism is not a treatment option of OEP analysis, because a prism prescription is viewed as treating a symptom rather than treating the underlying disorder.[12]

Another assumption in OEP analysis is that the standard OEP testing routine has been used. In this testing routine tests have been assigned numbers, by which they are often referred to in the OEP literature. The OEP test numbers and expecteds are given in Table 16.1. The OEP expecteds are graphed in Figure 16.1. It may be noted that the OEP expecteds are very similar to Morgan's mean values. They are all within

Table 16.1

The Optometric Extension Program test numbers and expecteds. The near tests are performed with a test distance of 16 inches with the exception of test no. 19.

Test Number	Test Description	Expecteds
1	Ophthalmoscopy	
2	Ophthalmometry	
3	Habitual lateral phoria at distance	0.5 exo
13A	Habitual lateral phoria at near	6 exo
4	Distance retinoscopy	
5	Retinoscopy at 20 inches (50 cm)	
6	Retinoscopy at 40 inches (1 m)	
7	Subjective refraction: maximum plus to 20/20 minus visual acuity	
7A	Maximum plus to best distance visual acuity	
8	Lateral phoria at distance through #7 finding	0.5 exo
9	Base-out to first blur at distance	7 to 9
10	Base-out to break and recovery at distance	19/10 minimum
11	Base-in to break and recovery at distance	9/5 minimum
12	Vertical phoria and fusional vergence ranges at distance	orthophoria, ranges equal
13B	Lateral phoria at near through no. #7 finding	6 exo
14A	Unfused (monocular) cross-cylinder	
15A	Lateral phoria at near through #14A finding	
14B	Fused (binocular) cross-cylinder	
15B	Lateral phoria at near through #14B finding	
16A	Base-out to blur-out at near	15
16B	Base-out to break and recovery at near	21/15 (minimum)
17A	Base-in to blur-out at near	14
17B	Base-in to break and recovery at near	22/18 (minimum)
18	Vertical phoria and fusional vergence ranges at near	orthophoria, ranges equal
19	Analytical amplitude (minus to blur of 0.62 m or J4 letters with card at 13 inches)	
20	Minus to blur-out	−2.25 to −2.50
21	Plus to blur-out	+1.75 to +2.00

one or two prism diopters of Morgan's means except the near phoria and the base-in and base-out recoveries at near. The plus-to-blur and minus-to-blur are essentially the same in the OEP expecteds and Morgan's mean values.

The analysis procedure begins with determining the case type. The case type is identified as A, B1, B2, or C through a procedure called "checking, chaining, and typing." These steps are (1) check: determine whether findings are high or low by comparing them with the expecteds;

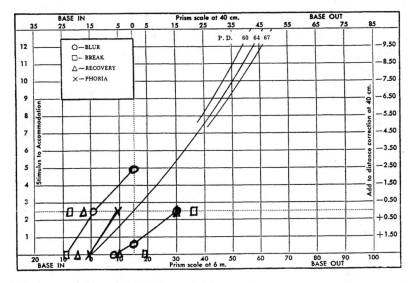

Figure 16.1 Plot of the OEP expecteds.

(2) chain: list the test numbers in a particular sequence above a horizontal line if they are high and below the line if they are low; and (3) type: use the "informative sequence" from checking and chaining to determine the case type.

The characteristic patterns of high and low findings for each of the case types are as follows:

A:

$$\overline{4 - 11 - 13B - 17B}$$

B1:

$$\frac{5}{9 - 11 - 16B}$$

B2:

$$\frac{5}{9 - 11 - 17B}$$

C:

$$\frac{15A}{5 - 10 - 16B}$$

The vast majority of cases are either B1 or B2 cases. Convergence insufficiency, pseudoconvergence insufficiency, and basic exo cases are usually typed B1, and convergence excess cases are usually typed B2. The remainder of the tests in the informative sequence are used to identify seven subtypes or "deteriorations" of B cases.

A series of rules are then applied to determine the lens prescription. The maximum plus prescribed for distance is the #7 finding, which is the point in the subjective refraction at which plus has been reduced to the level at which the patient can read most of the 20/20 line. The maximum plus prescribed for near is based on a formula that includes the #14B, #15B, and #19 test results. In B1 cases, full maximum plus is recommended for distance and near. In B2 cases, the directive is to prescribe the full plus at near but cut plus at distance. In C cases, the mandate is to cut plus at distance and near.

In OEP analysis the #16A, #17A, #20, and #21 findings are referred to as "equilibrium findings." Calculations are done to determine what these tests would yield if started at different levels of plus. An OEP directive is that the plus prescribed should not be so much that the equilibrium findings would be reversed from the habitual. In other words, if the #21 with the habitual correction is greater in magnitude than the #20, the plus prescribed should not be so high that the #20 becomes greater in magnitude than the #21.

Some findings also are used to establish a stage of embeddedness of a vision problem. There are directives concerning lens acceptance at different stages of embeddedness, with nonembedded cases thought to be more likely to accept plus lens application. Further information on OEP testing and analysis can be obtained from various sources.[10–16] The OEP uses a unique terminology, and the OEP literature that uses the vernacular can be difficult to understand. The easiest description to understand is that by Birnbaum.[12]

PRATT'S PLOTTING OF PHORIA AND BINOCULAR CROSS-CYLINDER LINES

Various investigators[17–19] have discussed systems for plotting ACA and CAC lines and for using this information for clinical analysis. Laboratory accommodative convergence and disparity-induced accommodation data have been plotted on the graph.[20,21] Pratt was perhaps the first to use such plots for clinical analysis.[22]

Pratt plotted phoria, binocular cross-cylinder (BCC), fusional vergence range, and relative accommodation data with accommodation in diopters on the x-axis and convergence in meter angles on the y-axis.

He measured phorias at 40 cm with various plus and minus adds, and did the BCC test at 40 cm through different base-in and base-out prism settings. The average data derived by Pratt are plotted in Figure 16.2 on coordinates like he used and in Figure 16.3 on the more familiar graph form.[22] The phoria and BCC lines cross at about the 1D point on the demand line on the average. The lateral placements and slopes of the phoria and BCC lines vary from patient to patient, but the BCC line always has a steeper slope when convergence is on the y-axis (Figure 16.2) and the phoria line has the steeper slope when accommodation is on the y-axis (Figure 16.3).

If Pratt found that for a given patient the BCC line was farther from the demand line than the phoria line, he prescribed a plus add. The power of the plus add was equal to the displacement in diopters on the x-axis from the 2.5-m angle point on the demand line to the point that was midway between the phoria and BCC lines at the level of 2.5-m angles on the y-axis. If the phoria line was farther from the demand line than the BCC line, Pratt prescribed a base in prism. The power of the

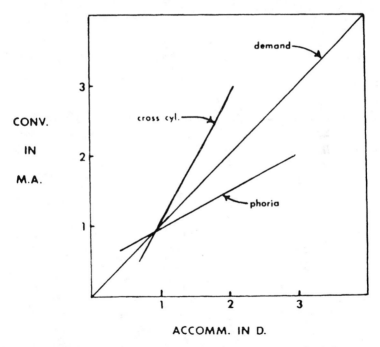

Figure 16.2 Average phoria and BCC data from Pratt plotted on the coordinates he used.

(Reprinted with permission from Goss DA. Pratt system of clinical analysis of accommodation and convergence. *Optom Vis Sci.* 1989;66:805–806. © The American Academy of Optometry. 1989.)

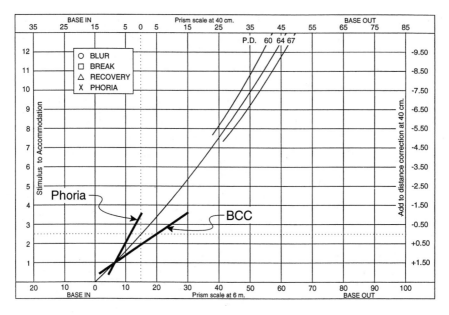

Figure 16.3 Average phoria and BCC data from Pratt plotted on the more familiar graph form.

(Reprinted with permission from Goss DA. Pratt system of clinical analysis of accommodation and convergence. *Optom Vis Sci.* 1989;66:805–806. © The American Academy of Optometry. 1989.)

base in prism was equal to the distance on the y-axis from the 2.5D point on the demand line to the point midway between the phoria and BCC lines at the level of 2.5D on the x-axis.

COMPARISON OF ACA AND CAC RATIOS

Schor and others[17–19,23–29] have discussed the clinical implications of the model of dual interactions of accommodation and convergence. In this model, if either the ACA or the CAC ratio is high without the other being low, there will be a binocular disorder. Take, for example, a case in which the ACA ratio is high, as in convergence excess, and the CAC ratio is average. As a result of the high ACA ratio, negative fusional vergence is required. The convergence accommodation change associated with negative fusional vergence is a decrease in accommodation. If the CAC ratio is not low, there will then need to be an increase in optical reflex accommodation to compensate for the decrease from convergence accommodation. This accommodation produces accommodative convergence and so on, back and forth between accommodative convergence and convergence accommodation.

The stopping point of these interactions leaves accommodation and vergence errors in the form of lag of accommodation and fixation disparity, respectively. Schor and Narayan[17] recommend correcting these errors with spherical lens adds (for convergence accommodation errors) or with prism (for accommodative convergence errors). The prism prescription should be equal to the associated phoria.

Schor and colleagues[17,23,24,27,28] include prism adaptation and accommodative adaptation in this model. Adaptation serves to reduce the interactions of accommodation and vergence. As prism adaptation replaces fusional vergence over a period of seconds or minutes, the amount of convergence accommodation is reduced. Likewise, accommodative adaptation reduces the lag of accommodation. Some vision training procedures may serve to improve the prism adaptation capabilities of an individual and are thus recommended in cases of accommodation and vergence interaction disorders.

Daum et al[19] reported a study assessing a diagnostic criterion similar to Sheard's criterion, but based on the interaction model. They presented a graphical method and a formula for determining the fusional demand under binocular conditions. They determined a CAC ratio with Nott retinoscopy with the target at 40 cm using varying amounts of prism to change the level of convergence. An example of their graph is shown in Figure 16.4. The ACA line was drawn through the phoria points. The CAC line was plotted with a slope equal to the CAC ratio through the 40-cm demand line point. The lateral displacement of the intersection of these lines from the demand line point for 40 cm represented the demand on vergence under binocular conditions due to the interactions of accommodative convergence and convergence accommodation. The formula for the demand on vergence under binocular conditions (DV) is:

$$DV = (CR - (AR \times ACA))/(1 - (ACA \times CAC))$$

where CR is the convergence response from both accommodative convergence and fusional convergence, AR is the accommodative response from both blur-driven accommodation and convergence accommodation, ACA is the ACA ratio, and CAC is the CAC ratio. DV was then used as the demand value in the classical Sheard's criterion formula.

Daum et al[19] examined 100 subjects to test the effectiveness of this new criterion in distinguishing symptomatic from asymptomatic individuals. The new criterion correctly distinguished six subjects more than the classical Sheard's criterion, but stepwise discriminant analysis did not show superiority of the calculated fusional demand or the new criterion over the near phoria or the classical Sheard's criterion value.

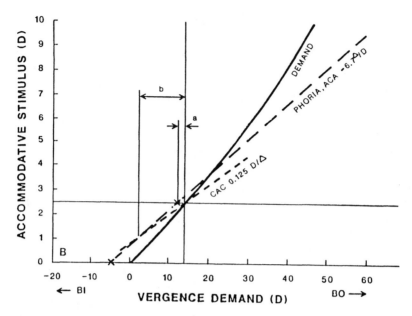

Figure 16.4 An example of the plot of ACA and CAC lines used by Daum et al. The subject whose data are portrayed here had a distance dissociated phoria of 4Δ exophoria and a near dissociated phoria of 2Δ exophoria. The letter a represents the magnitude of the near dissociated phoria. The letter b represents the magnitude of the vergence imbalance predicted by interactions of accommodative convergence and convergence accommodation.

(Reprinted with permission from Daum KM, Rutstein RP, Houston G IV, Clore KA, Corliss DA. Evaluation of a new criterion of binocularity. *Optom Vis Sci.* 1989;66:218–228. © The American Academy of Optometry, 1989.)

These investigators suggested that further development of the procedure is needed.

REFERENCES

1. Griffin, JR. Binocular Anomalies—Procedures for Vision Therapy. 2nd ed. New York, NY: Professional Press; 1982:335–344, 378–411.
2. Grisham JD. Treatment of binocular dysfunctions. In: Schor CM, Ciuffreda KJ, eds. *Vergence Eye Movements: Basic and Clinical Aspects.* Boston, MA: Butterworth-Heinemann; 1983:605–646.
3. Cooper J. Accommodative dysfunction. In: Amos JF, ed. *Diagnosis and Management in Vision Care.* Boston, MA: Butterworths; 1987:431–459.
4. Wick BC. Horizontal deviations. In: Amos JF, ed. *Diagnosis and Management in Vision Care.* Boston, MA: Butterworth-Heinemann; 1983:461–513.

5. Grosvenor TP. *Primary Care Optometry*. 2nd ed. Boston, MA: Butterworth-Heinemann; 1989:96–110, 338–352.

6. Scheiman M, Wick B. *Clinical Management of Binocular Vision—Heterophoric, Accommodative, and Eye Movement Disorders*. Philadelphia, PA: Lippincott; 1994: 219–378.

7. Saladin JJ. Horizontal prism prescription. In: Cotter SA, ed. *Clinical Uses of Prism— A Spectrum of Applications—Mosby's Optometric Problem Solving Series*. St Louis, MO: Mosby-Year Book. 1995:109–147.

8. Borish IM. *Clinical Refraction*. 3rd ed. Boston, MA: Butterworth-Heinemann; 1970:861–937.

9. Birnbaum MH. *Optometric Management of Nearpoint Vision Disorders*. Boston, MA: Butterworth-Heinemann; 1993:33–71.

10. Manas L. *Visual Analysis*. 3rd ed. Chicago, IL: Professional Press; 1965.

11. Margach CB. *Introduction to Functional Optometry*. Duncan, OK: Optometric Extension Program Foundation; 1979.

12. Birnbaum MH. *Optometric Management of Nearpoint Vision Disorders*. Boston, MA: Butterworth-Heinemann; 1993:121–160.

13. Dvorine I. *Theory and Practice of Analytical Refraction and Orthoptics*. Baltimore, MA: French-Bray; 1948.

14. Lesser SK. *Introduction to Modern Analytical Optometry*. Revised ed. Duncan, OK: Optometric Extension Program; 1969.

15. Slade GC. *Modern Clinical Optometry—A Guide and Review*. Duncan, OK: Optometric Extension Program; 1972.

16. Pheiffer CH. *Analytical Analysis of A.M. Skeffington and Associates*. Duncan, OK: Optometric Extension Program Foundation; 1981.

17. Schor CM, Narayan B. Graphical analysis of prism adaptation, convergence accommodation, and accommodative convergence. *Am J Optom Physiol Opt.* 1982;59:774–784.

18. Wick B, London R. Analysis of binocular visual function using tests made under binocular conditions. *Am J Optom Physiol Opt.* 1987;64:227–240.

19. Daum KM, Rutstein RP, Houston G IV, Clore KA, Corliss DA. Evaluation of a new criterion of binocularity. *Optom Vis Sci.* 1989;66:218–228.

20. Fincham EF, Walton J. The reciprocal actions of accommodation and convergence. *J Physiol.* 1957;137:488–508.

21. Balsam MH, Fry GA. Convergence accommodation. *Am J Optom Arch Am Acad Optom.* 1959;36:567–575.

22. Goss DA. Pratt system of clinical analysis of accommodation and convergence. *Optom Vis Sci.* 1989;66:805–806.

23. Schor CM. Fixation disparity and vergence adaptation. In: Schor CM, Ciuffreda KJ, eds. *Vergence Eye Movements: Basic and Clinical Aspects*. Boston, MA: Butterworth-Heinemann; 1983:465–516.

24. Schor CM. Analysis of tonic and accommodative vergence disorders of binocular vision. *Am J Optom Physiol Opt.* 1983;60:1–14.

25. Wick B. Clinical factors in proximal vergence. *Am J Optom Physiol Opt.* 1985;62:1–18.

26. Saladin JJ. Interpretation of divergent oculomotor imbalance through control system analysis. *Am J Optom Physiol Opt.* 1988;65:439–447.

27. Schor C. Influence of accommodative and vergence adaptation on binocular motor disorders. *Am J Optom Physiol Opt.* 1988;65:464–475.

28. Schor C, Horner D. Adaptive disorders of accommodation and vergence in binocular dysfunction. *Ophthal Physiol Opt.* 1989;9:264–268.
29. Scheiman M, Wick B. *Clinical Management of Binocular Vision—Heterophoric, Accommodative, and Eye Movement Disorders.* Philadelphia, PA: Lippincott; 1994: 469–489.

SUGGESTED READING

Birnbaum MH. *Optometric Management of Nearpoint Vision Disorders.* Boston, MA: Butterworth-Heinemann; 1993:128–168.
Saladin JJ. Horizontal prism prescription. In: Cotter SA, ed. *Clinical Uses of Prism— A Spectrum of Applications—Mosby's Optometric Problem Solving Series.* St. Louis, MO: Mosby-Year Book: 1995: 109–147.
Scheiman M, Wick B. *Clinical Management of Binocular Vision-Heterophorid, Accommodative, and Eye Movement Disorders.* Philadelphia, PA: Lippincott; 1994: 476–485.

17

Vertical Imbalances

Vertical imbalances, as well as horizontal imbalances, may be a cause of visual complaints. The person with a vertical phoria may complain of a pulling sensation, headaches, asthenopia, skipping lines or losing place when reading, and/or diplopia, especially a diplopia in which the images are one above the other. In the presence of such complaints and the absence of other obvious causes, the optometrist should carefully watch for a vertical movement on the cover test and should measure the dissociated vertical phoria,[1] perhaps in more than one way to check the validity of the measurements. In addition to the von Graefe technique in the phoropter, the dissociated phoria can be taken by means of the Maddox rod, the stereoscope, or other methods. Vertical-dissociated phorias measured by different instruments or at various distances usually will not differ significantly. If the vertical dissociated phoria is not zero, the vertical associated phoria (vertical prism, which reduces the vertical fixation disparity to zero) should be tested. Because accommodative convergence does not affect vertical phorias, spherical lens adds are not used to treat a primary vertical imbalance. The treatment of choice for vertical imbalances is vertical prism. A less commonly used option is vision training. Some hints and guidelines for handling vertical imbalances are given in this chapter.

In cases of high refractive error, it is important that there be no tilt of the phoropter or of the spectacles, so that a vertical phoria is not induced by the lenses. One way to solve this problem in the phoropter is to align the patient so that the target is seen through the pinholes and then to repeat the phoria.

The vertical fusional amplitudes can be used as a check on the dissociated vertical phoria. Borish[2] suggests the use of the following formula:

$$\frac{\text{Base-down to break} - \text{Base-up to break}}{2} = \text{Correcting prism}$$

If the resultant correcting prism value is positive, base-down is indicated; if negative, base-up is indicated. Borish suggests that when the imbalance indicated by the phoria and the imbalance indicated by the vertical fusional amplitudes disagree, the value prescribed should be the prism that equalizes the fusional amplitudes, as given in the formula. The vertical phoria may differ from the vertical fusional amplitude imbalance as a result of the lateral vergence difference during the two types of measurement.

Some clinicians recommend vision training to try to provide comfortable binocular vision to patients with vertical phorias, even though the prescription of some prism may be necessary after the completion of the training program. Wick and Scheiman[3,4] described a training program for vertical phorias in which horizontal vergence training, vertical vergence training, and antisuppression training are combined.

Vertical prism adaptation has been described by many investigators.[5-11] Patients with effective prism adaptation are usually asymptomatic. In general, vertical prism should not be prescribed for asymptomatic patients.

Although vertical fixation disparity curves are not used as commonly as horizontal fixation disparity curves, they can be plotted using an instrument such as the Disparometer. Vertical fixation disparity also can be determined with the Wesson fixation disparity card by rotating the card 90 degrees so that the fixation disparity lines are horizontal. Most vertical fixation disparity curves are best fitted by a straight line.[12] The vertical associated phoria is the vertical prism that reduces the vertical fixation disparity to zero. It can be measured with devices such as the Mallett unit, Bernell lantern-associated phoria unit, AO vectographic slide, or Borish card (see Chapter 10). The x-intercept on the vertical fixation disparity curve is also a measurement of the associated phoria. There seems to be unanimous opinion that the vertical associated phoria is the best way to prescribe vertical prism.[4,8,13-19] If the vertical associated phoria is zero, no prism prescription is indicated. The prism prescription should be equal to the associated phoria. Prism prescribed in this way, even as little as one or sometimes one-half prism diopter, often will be effective in relieving the symptoms of vertical phorias. Rutstein and Eskridge[12] suggested that in prescribing vertical prism, it is important to measure associated phorias at distance and near in straight-ahead and down-gaze.

Borish[2] reports a subjective technique for evaluating the acceptance of vertical prism. The technique consists of having the patient view letters of best visual acuity at both distance and near, with the proposed prism in a trial fame, and requesting the patient to indicate whether there is an improvement in visual acuity or a subjective feeling of relief. The prism can then be oriented in other directions and the steps repeated to test the possibility of the prism simply having a placebo effect. If the prism is subjectively agreeable to the patient only with the base oriented the same as in the original measurement, it should be prescribed.

In summary, a vertical imbalance should be corrected with prism (1) whenever it is accompanied by significant ocular symptoms, (2) when the testing techniques give consistent results, (3) when the dissociated vertical phoria is correlated with a vertical fixation disparity in the same direction, and (4) when there is an absence of significant prism adaptation. Associated phorias should be used as the basis for prescribing vertical prism power.

REFERENCES

1. Daum KM. Heterophoria and heterotropia. In: Eskridge JB, Amos JF, Bartlett JD, eds. *Clinical Procedures in Optometry.* Philadelphia, PA: Lippincott; 1991:72–90.
2. Borish IM. *Clinical Refraction.* 3rd ed. Boston, MA: Butterworth-Heinemann; 1970:872–873.
3. Wick B. Vision therapy for cyclovertical heterophoria. In: London R, ed. Ocular Vertical and Cyclovertical Deviations. *Probl Optometry.* 1992;4:652–66.
4. Scheiman M, Wick B. *Clinical Management of Binocular Vision—Heterophoric, Accommodative, and Eye Movement Disorders.* Philadelphia, PA: Lippincott; 1994: 405–440.
5. Ellerbrock V, Fry GA. The after-effect induced by vertical divergence. *Am J Optom Arch Am Acad Optom.* 1941;18:450–454.
6. Ellerbrock VJ. Tonicity induced by fusional movements. *Am J Optom Arch Am Acad Optom.* 1950;27:8–20.
7. Carter DB. Effects of prolonged wearing of prism. *Am J Optom Arch Am Acad Optom.* 1963;40:265–273.
8. Sheedy JE. *Fixation Disparity Curves.* Columbus, OH: Vision Analysis; 1979:7–8.
9. Henson DB, North R. Adaptation to prism-induced heterophoria. *Am J Optom Physiol Opt.* 1980;57:129–137.
10. Rutstein RP, Eskridge JB. Clinical evaluation of vertical fixation disparity. Part III. Adaptation to vertical prism. *Am J Optom Physiol Opt.* 1985;62:585–590.
11. Eskridge JB. Vertical muscle adaptation. In: London R, ed. Ocular Vertical and Cyclovertical Deviations. *Probl Optometry.* 1992;4:622–628.
12. Rutstein RP, Eskridge JB. Clinical evaluation of vertical fixation disparity. Part one. *Am J Optom Physiol Opt.* 1983;60:688–693.
13. Mallett RFJ. Fixation disparity in clinical practice. *Aust J Optom.* 1969;52: 97–109.
14. Grosvenor T. Clinical use of fixation disparity. *Optom Weekly.* 1975;66: 1224–1228.
15. Eskridge JB, Rutstein RP. Clinical evaluation of vertical fixation disparity. Part IV. Slope and adaptation to vertical prism of vertical heterophoria patients. *Am J Optom Physiol Opt.* 1986;63:662–667.
16. Rutstein RP, Eskridge JB. Studies in vertical fixation disparity. *Am J Optom Physiol Opt.* 1986;63:639–644.
17. Amos JF, Rutstein RP. Vertical deviations. In: Amos JF, ed. *Diagnosis and Management in Vision Care.* Boston, MA: Butterworth-Heinemann; 1987: 515–583.
18. Cotter SA, Frantz KA. Prescribing prism for vertical deviations. In: London R, ed. Ocular Vertical and Cyclovertical Deviations. *Probl Optometry.* 1992;4: 629–645.

19. Wick B. Prescribing prism for patients with vertical heterophoria. In: Cotter, SA, ed. *Clinical Uses of Prism–A Spectrum of Applications—Mosby's Optometric Problem Solving Series.* St. Louis, MO: Mosby-Year Book; 1995:149–175.

SUGGESTED READING

Amos JF, Rutstein RP. Vertical deviations. In: Amos JF, ed. *Diagnosis and Management in Vision Care.* Boston, MA: Butterworth-Heinemann; 1987:515–583.

London R, ed. Ocular vertical and cyclovertical deviations. *Probl Optometry.* 1992;4:541–683.

Rutstein RP, Eskridge JB. Studies in vertical fixation disparity. *Am J Optom Physiol Opt.* 1986;63:639–644.

Appendix A

Answers to Practice Problems

Answers to selected practice problems given at the end of the chapters:

Chapter 1

1. 80 cm: 1.25D

   75 cm: 1.33D

   45 cm: 2.22D

   36 cm: 2.78D

   30 cm: 3.33D

   15 cm: 6.67D

Chapter 2

1.

PATIENT AD:

Calculated ACA ratio $= \dfrac{16.7 - (-1) + (-2)}{3.00} = 5.2\Delta/D$

PATIENT EJ:

Gradient ACA ratio $= 3\Delta/D$

Calculated ACA ratio $= \dfrac{15 - (1) + (-4)}{2.50} = 4\Delta/D$

PATIENT TB:

Calculated ACA ratio $= \dfrac{15 - 0 + (-2)}{2.50} = 5.2\Delta/D$

Calculated ACA ratio $= \dfrac{17.8 - 0 + (-2)}{3.00} = 5.3\Delta/D$

PATIENT SP:

Calculated ACA ratio $= \dfrac{15.7 - 2 + 4}{2.50} = 7.1\Delta/D$

PATIENT GP:

Calculated ACA ratio $= \dfrac{14.8 - 0 + (-9)}{2.50} = 2.3\Delta/D$

2. ACA ratios calculated from Figure 2.1, assuming 64-mm PD:

Gradient ACA ratio $= 3\Delta/D$

Calculated ACA ratio $= \dfrac{15 - 0 + (-5)}{2.5} = 4.0\Delta/D$

Calculated ACA ratio $= \dfrac{17.8 - 0 + (-6)}{3.00} = 3.9\Delta/D$

Calculated ACA ratio $= \dfrac{15 - 0 + (-8)}{1.50} = 4.7\Delta/D$

ACA ratios calculated from Figure 2.2, assuming 64-mm PD:

ACA ratio $= \dfrac{15 - (-1) + 5}{2.50} = 8.4\Delta/D$

ACA ratio $= \dfrac{17.8 - (-1) + 6}{3.00} = 8.3\Delta/D$

ACA ratio $= \dfrac{15 - (-1) + (-3)}{1.50} = 8.7\Delta/D$

ACA ratio calculated from Figure 2.3, assuming 64-mm PD:

ACA ratio $= \dfrac{15 - 0 + 0}{2.5} = 6.0\Delta/D$

Chapter 3

PATIENT BP

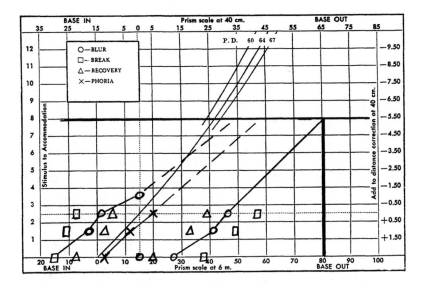

No findings appear erroneous.

Gradient ACA ratio = 8Δ/D

Calculated ACA ratio $= \dfrac{14.5 - 2 + 5}{2.50} = 7Δ/D$

PATIENT AT:

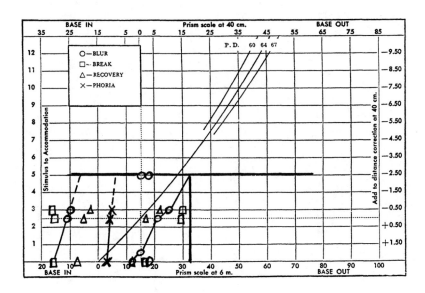

33 cm plus-to-blur appears erroneous.

$$\text{Calculated ACA ratio} = \frac{15.5 - (-3) + (-11)}{2.50} = 3\Delta/D$$

$$\text{Calculated ACA ratio} = \frac{18.3 - (-3) + (-13)}{3.00} = 2.8\Delta/D$$

PATIENT GP:

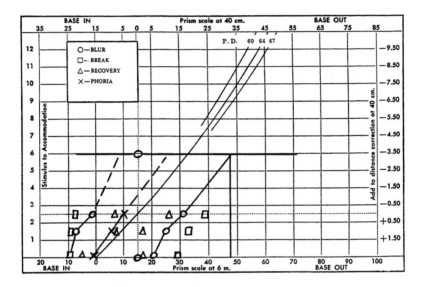

No findings appear erroneous.

Gradient ACA ratio = $4\Delta/D$

$$\text{Calculated ACA ratio} = \frac{15 - (-1) + (-5)}{2.50} = 4.4\Delta/D$$

PATIENT DK:

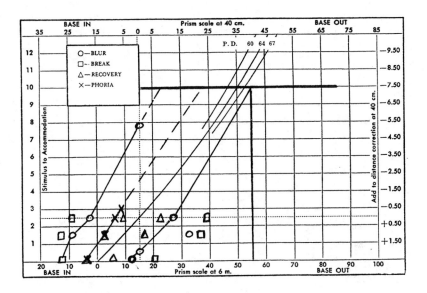

40 cm + 1.00 add, base-out blur, appears erroneous.

Gradient ACA ratio = 4Δ/D

Calculated ACA ratio = $\dfrac{15 - (-4) + (-8)}{2.50}$ = 4.4Δ/D

Calculated ACA ratio = $\dfrac{17.8 - (-4) + (-9)}{3.00}$ = 4.3Δ/D

PATIENT HF:

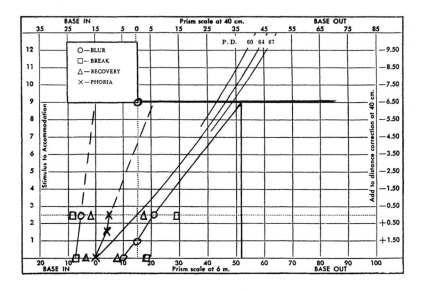

No findings appear erroneous.

Gradient ACA ratio = 1Δ/D

Calculated ACA ratio = $\dfrac{14 - 0 + (-10)}{2.50}$ = 1.6Δ/D

Chapter 5

	Patient BP	Patient AT	Patient GP	Patient DK	Patient HF
6 m					
NRC	15	16	10	12	8
PRC	28	12	20	12	10
NFC	17	13	9	8	8
PFC	26	15	21	16	10
NFRC	15	*	*	*	*
PFRC	*	12	10	12	*
40 cm					
NRC	14	26	16	18	20
PRC	32	6	16	12	6

	Patient BP	Patient AT	Patient GP	Patient DK	Patient HF
NFC	19	15	11	10	10
PFC	27	17	21	20	16
NFRC	14	*	*	*	*
PFRC	*	6	16	12	6
NRA	+2.50	+2.00	+2.50	+2.00	+1.50
PRA	−1.00	−2.50	−3.50	−5.25	−6.50

*Does not apply.

Chapter 7

		Patient GH	Patient JK	Patient RP	Patient LP	Patient MS
1		12 2/3	10 2/3	12 2/3	9 1/3	10
2		2	12	5	8	6
3	NRC	14	28	14	20	6
	PRC	24	4	24	8	24
	NFC	12	16	19	12	12
	PFC	26	16	19	16	18
4		24	4	14	8	6
5	Calculated ACA	5.9Δ/D	2.8Δ/D, 2.3Δ/D	8.1Δ/D	2.2Δ/D	6.4Δ/D
	Gradient ACA	3Δ/D	———	9Δ/D	2Δ/D	5Δ/D
6a	Prism Lens	Yes	No 1 1/3Δ base-in −0.48D	Yes	Yes	Yes
	VT		Increase base-out to 8Δ			
6b	Prism Lens	Yes	No 6 2/3Δ base-in −2.38D	Yes	No 2 2/3Δ base-in −1.34D	No 2Δ base-out +0.40D
	VT		Increase base-out to 24Δ		Increase base-out to 16Δ	Increase base-in to 12Δ

		Patient GH	Patient JK	Patient RP	Patient LP	Patient MS
7a	Distance	Yes	No	Yes	Yes	Yes
	Prism		2 2/3Δ base-in			
	Lens		-0.95D			
	VT		Increase base-out to 8Δ			
7b	Near	Yes	No	Yes	No	No
	Prism		6 2/3Δ base-in		1 1/3Δ base-in	4Δ base-out
	Lens		-2.38D		-0.67D	+0.80D
	VT		Increase base-out to 14Δ		Increase base-out to 10Δ	Increase base-in to 12Δ
8a	Distance	Does not apply	Does not apply	Does not apply	Yes	No
	Prism					1Δ base-out
	Lens					—
	VT					Increase base-in recovery to 4Δ
8b	Near	Does not apply	Does not apply	Yes	Does not apply	No
	Prism					1.5Δ base-out
	Lens					+0.30D
	VT					Increase base-in recovery to 6Δ

Chapter 8

1.

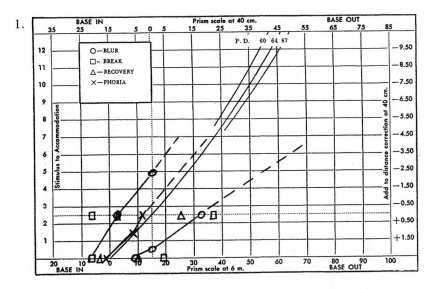

2.

$$\text{Calculated ACA ratio} = \frac{15 - (-1) + (-3)}{2.50} = 5.2\Delta/D$$

The calculated ACA ratio is greater than the gradient ACA ratio because the calculated ACA ratio includes proximal convergence and the gradient does not.

3. The positive width of the zone (PFC) at 40 cm is 20Δ. The negative width of the zone (NFC) is 10Δ. The positive width is greater.

4. a. near phoria
   b. base-out fusional amplitudes

Chapter 10

3. Patient JS

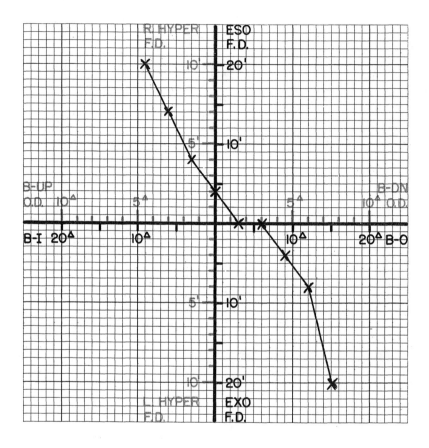

Patient CR

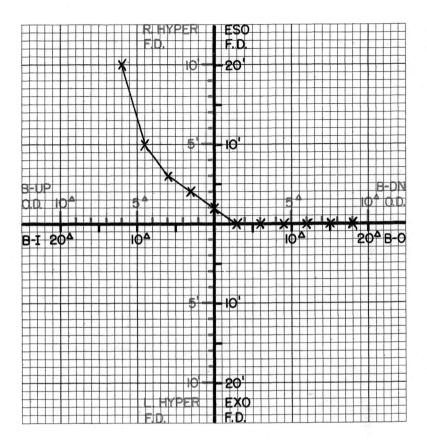

Patient JB

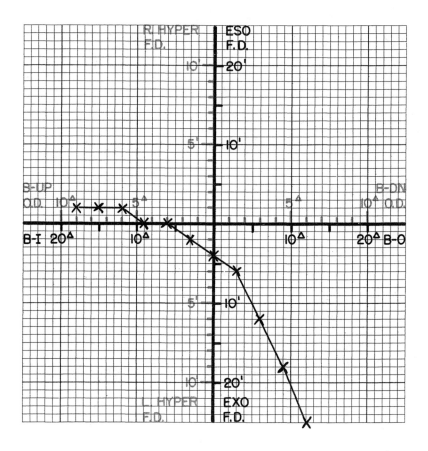

Patient RM

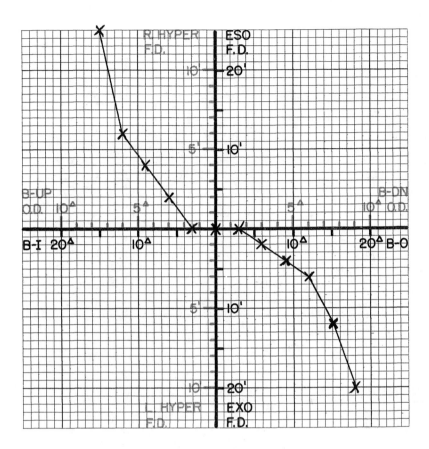

	Patient JS	Patient CR	Patient JB	Patient RM
Curve type	I	II	III	I
Slope	$-1.3'/\Delta$	$-0.7'/\Delta$	$-0.7'/\Delta$	0
y-intercept	4′ eso	2′ eso	4′ exo	0
x-intercept	3Δ base-out	3Δ base-out	6Δ base-in	0
Center of symmetry	3Δ base-out	3Δ base-out	6Δ base-in	0

Chapter 11

PATIENT PR

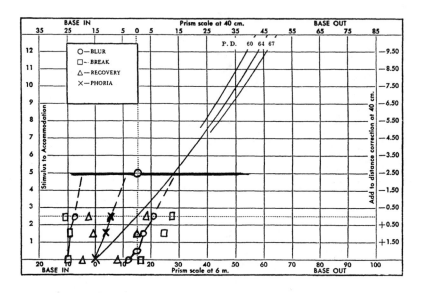

PATIENT ST

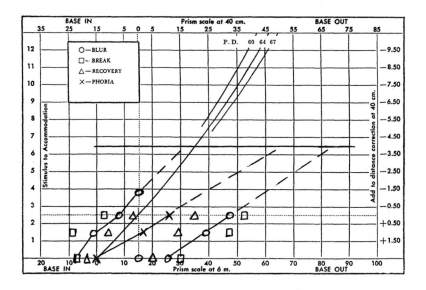

PATIENT RK

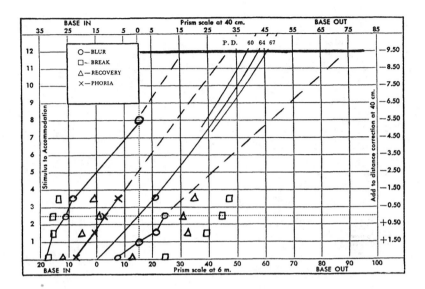

PATIENT EN

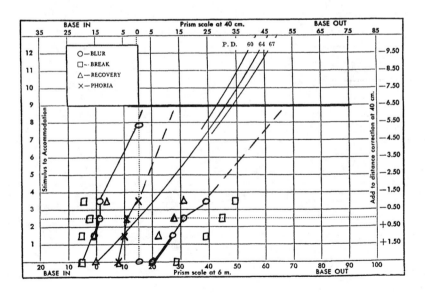

PATIENT CD

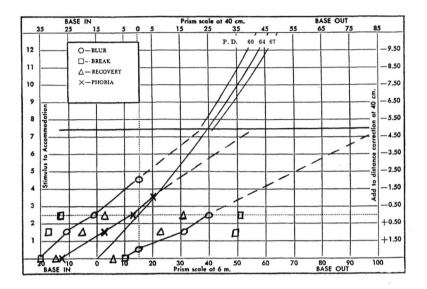

	Patient PR	Patient ST	Patient RK	Patient EN	Patient CD
+1.00 D Gradient ACA ratio	2ΔD	10	4	1	10
Calculated ACA ratio	2.4ΔD	10.8	4	1	10.1
Sheard's criterion at distance	Met	Met	Not met	Not met	Not met
Sheard's criterion at near	Not met	Not met	Not met	Met	Met
Percival's criterion at distance	Met	Not met	Not met	Not met	Met
Percival's criterion at near	Not met	Not met	Not met	Met	Met
Case type	Convergence insufficiency	Convergence excess	Basic Esophoria	Divergence insufficiency	Divergence excess

Chapter 12

PATIENT EB:
1. +2.00D

2. +1.75D

Calculated ACA ratio $= \dfrac{15 - (-1) + (-14)}{2.50 - 2.00} = 4\Delta/D$

Calculated ACA ratio $= \dfrac{17.8 - (-1) + (-15)}{3.00 - 2.00} = 3.8\Delta/D$

PATIENT TC:
1. +1.40D (rounded to +1.25D or +1.50D)

2. Judging from the graph, +1.00D to +1.25D

3.

Calculated ACA ratio $= \dfrac{15 - 0 + (-9)}{2.50 - 1.25} = 4.8\Delta/D$

Calculated ACA ratio $= \dfrac{17.8 - 0 + (-10)}{3.00 - 1.25} = 4.4\Delta/D$

PATIENT JF:
1. +1.00D

2. +1.00D

Calculated ACA ratio $= \dfrac{15 - 1 + 1}{2.50 - 1.00} = 10\Delta/D$

Calculated ACA ratio $= \dfrac{15 - 1 + (-5)}{2.50 - 1.50} = 9\Delta/D$

PATIENT CB:
1. + 1.25D

2. + 1.00D

3.

Calculated ACA ratio $= \dfrac{15 - (-2) + (-12)}{2.50 - 1.00} = 3.3\Delta/D$

Calculated ACA ratio $= \dfrac{15 - (-2) + (-14)}{2.50 - 1.50} = 3\Delta/D$

Chapter 13

1. Minimum expected amplitude = 15 − (0.25) (20) = 10D. This condition would be called "accommodative insufficiency." Potential treatments are a plus add and/or vision training.

2. CD: accommodative response = 2.08D; lag of accommodation = 0.42D
   GI: accommodative response = 1.47D; lag of accommodation = 1.03D
   FC: accommodative response = 1.79D; lag of accommodation = 0.71D

   Patient GI has a higher than normal lag of accommodation. The usual treatment is a plus add for near.

3. The lag of accommodation is 1.25D, which is higher than normal.

4. Lens rock includes optical cues. Distance rock includes both optical and proximal cues. The change in distance on the distance rock test provides proximal cues.

Chapter 15

7. Patient BL:
   b.

   $$\text{Calculated ACA ratio} = \frac{15 - (-10) + (-16)}{2.50} = 3.6\Delta/D$$

   c. All distances
   d. Orthotropia could be achieved with minus lens additions

8. Patient DM:

   a. Inside approximately 50 cm
   b. All distances, because the accommodative convergence which occurs when the hyperopia is uncorrected increases the amount of eso.
   c.

   $$\text{Calculated ACA ratio} = \frac{15 - 7 + 17}{2.50} = 10\Delta/D$$

   Gradient ACA ratio = 10Δ/D

   d. Treatment for this patient would include full correction of the hyperopia and a plus add for near, as well as base-out prism and/or vision training to improve negative fusional vergence.

Appendix B

Equipment Sources

The American Optical Vectographic Slide (Figure 10.1) and the Bernell lantern with distance (Figure 10.2) and near (Figure 10.4) associated phoria targets are available from Bernell Corporation, 750 Lincolnway East, PO Box 4637, South Bend, IN 46634–4637; customer service telephone (219)234–3200.

The Mallett units for distance (Figure 10.3) and near (Figures 10.5 and 10.6) associated phoria testing are available from Optec International Ltd, 20 Glenmere Ave, Mill Hill, London NW 7 2LU, England; telephone 081–959–1279.

The Sheedy Disparometer (Figures 10.8 and 10.9) is available from Vision Analysis, 136 Hillcroft Way, Walnut Creek, CA 94596.

The Wesson Fixation Disparity Card (Figure 10.10) is available from Dr Michael Wesson, 4912 Indian Valley Rd, Birmingham, AL 35244.

Lens rock accommodative facility flippers (Figure 13.1), the dynamic retinoscopy test card shown in Figure 13.2, Brock strings (Figure 14.3), vectograms (Figure 14.5) and tranaglyphs, Hart charts (Figure 14.10) for distance rock accommodative facility training, and a chiastopic fusion target (Figure 14.13, right) are available from Bernell Corporation, 750 Lincolnway East, PO Box 4637, South Bend, IN 46634–4637; customer service telephone (219)234–3200.

A chiastopic fusion card (Figure 14.13, left) is available from Mast/Keystone, 4637 Aircenter Circle, Reno, NV 89502; telephone (702)827–8110.

Index

Absolute presbyopia, 121
ACA ratio, 40, 176
    CAC ratio, comparison, 190–192
    calculated ACA ratio, 12, 176
    and convergence, 164–179
    drug effects, 172
    gradient ACA ratio, 47–48, 51, 176
    response ACA ratio, 34
    stability, 171–172
    stimulus ACA ratio, 12–13, 35
    strabismus, 179
    vergence disorders, 94–106
Accommodation
    amplitude of, 6, 22–23, 120–121
    convergence accommodation, 166,
        167–169
    disparity-induced accommodation,
        167
    lag of, 34–35, 137–141
    lead of, 137, 141
    near-point of accommodation, 22–23
    negative relative accommodation,
        43–45, 140
    optical reflex accommodation, 173,
        174
    paralysis of, 142
    positive relative accommodation,
        43–45, 97, 140
    proximal accommodation, 173
    stimulus to, 2–6
Accommodation insufficiency, 142, 143
Accommodative adaptation, 191
Accommodative convergence, 11, 12, 40
    ACA ratio, 171, 176
    fixation disparity, 73
    fusional ranges, 164
    lenses, 73
Accommodative disorders
    nonpresbyopic, 136–146
    presbyopia, 120–129
    vision training, 141, 150–161, 191
Accommodative excess, 142, 143
Accommodative facility, 135–136,
    156–157

Accommodative fatigue, 142, 143
Accommodative infacility, 142, 143
Accommodative insufficiency, 142, 143
Accommodative ranges, 123–124
Accommodative response, 34, 164
Accommodative rock, 141
Accommodative stimulus, 135, 137
Alpern, M., 171
Ametropia, 12
Amplitude of accommodation, 6,
    22–23, 120–121
Angle of anomaly, 179
Anomalous retinal correspondence, 179
Area of comfort, 53
Associated phoria, 70, 71, 109
Asthenopia, 69, 76, 84, 125, 177

Base-in prism, 9
Base-in to blur, break, and recovery, 6,
    21, 25, 51–52
Base-out prism, 9, 98–99, 103
Base-out to blur, break, and recovery,
    6, 21, 25
Basic esophoria, 103–105, 108
Basic exophoria, 101–103, 108
BCC. See Binocular cross-cylinder test
Bernell lantern, 78, 79, 217
Binocular cross-cylinder (BCC) test, 6,
    137, 139–140
    add correction, 122–123
    phoria, 188–190
Binocular lens rock test, 137
Binocular lens rock vision training,
    156
Binocular vision syndromes,
    13–15
Birnbaum, M. H., 177, 188
Borish, I. M., 185, 195, 196
Borish card, 79, 81
Brock string, 152–153, 217
Buzzelli, A. R., 175

CAC ratio, 166–167, 190–192
Calculated ACA ratio, 12

Carter, D. B., 107
Case type, OEP, 186
Checking, chaining, and typing, 186
Chiastopic fusion targets, vision training, 159–160, 217
Comfort zone, 53
Convergence, 11
  and accommodation, 164–179
  accommodative convergence, 11, 12, 40, 73, 164, 171, 176
  disparity convergence, 30
  fusional convergence, 11, 40, 73, 177
  near-point of, 6, 23, 95, 150–151
  negative fusional convergence, 41, 154–155
  negative fusional reserve convergence, 41, 47
  negative relative convergence, 41, 47, 97
  positive fusional convergence, 41, 69, 150–151, 154–155
  positive fusional reserve convergence, 41, 47
  positive relative convergence, 41, 47, 95
  proximal convergence, 11, 28–29, 35–38, 40, 171
  psychic convergence, 40
  tonic convergence, 11, 40
  triad convergence, 168
Convergence accommodation, 166, 167–169
Convergence amplitude, 23
Convergence disorders, vision training, 150–161
Convergence excess, 13–15, 94, 97–98, 108
Convergence insufficiency, 13–15, 56, 108
  false convergence insufficiency, 35
    see also pseudoconvergence insufficiency
  prescription, 95–96
  vision training, 160
Convergence stimulus, 2–6, 13
Cross, A. J., 139
Cross dynamic retinoscopy, 139

Dalziel, C. C., 47
Dark focus, 174

Dark vergence, 174
Daum, K. M., 167, 191
Delgadillo, H. M., 175
Demand line (Donders line), 2, 4, 175–177
Demand on vergence, 191–192
Depth of focus, 170
Divergence excess, 13–15, 94, 108
Diopter, 2, 173
Dioptric accommodative stimulus, 135, 137, 139
Disparity convergence, 30
Disparity-induced accommodation, 167
Disparometer, 68, 82–83, 196, 217
Dissociated phoria, 6, 9, 70, 71, 76
  fixation disparity, 69
  vertical imbalance, 195
Distance phoria, 11
Distance rock test, 135, 137
Distance rock vision training, 157–158, 217
Divergence excess, 13–15, 99–101
Divergence insufficiency, 13–15, 98–99, 108
Donders, F. C., 2, 121
Donders line (demand line), 2, 4, 175–177
Drug effects, 172
Duane, Alexander, 13, 121
Dynamic retinoscopy, 137–139, 140, 217

Embeddedness, 188
Equipment sources, 217
Erroneous findings, graphical analysis, 24–28
Eskridge, J. B., 196
Eso fixation disparity, 70, 74
Esophoria, 42, 43, 47, 50–51, 76, 85
  basic esophoria, 103–105, 108
  fixation disparity, 85
  prescription, 103–105
  Sheard's criterion, 47, 50–51
Ethyl alcohol, 172
Exo fixation disparity, 68, 70, 74
Exophoria, 9, 12, 42, 43, 47–50, 76, 85, 125
  basic exophoria, 101–103, 108
  fixation disparity, 85

Exophoria–*cont.*
  presbyopia, 125
  prescription, 101–103
  Sheard's criterion, 47–50

False convergence insufficiency, 35
  see also pseudoconvergence
    insufficiency
FDC. *See* Fixation disparity curve
Fixation disparity, 68–74, 76–87, 196
Fixation disparity curve (FDC), 70–73,
    76, 82–87
Focus
  dark focus, 174
  depth of, 170
Fry, G., 2, 168
Fusional aftereffects, 71, 171
Fusional amplitude, 178, 195
Fusional convergence, 11, 40
  asthenopia, 177
  fixation disparity, 73

Gilmartin, B., 174
Goss, D. A., 140
Gradient ACA ratio, 47–48, 51, 176
Graphical analysis, 1–7, 140, 175
  amplitude of accommodation,
    22–23
  base-in and base-out findings, 21
  convergence amplitude, 23
  erroneous findings, 24–28
  phorias, 9–15
  planning vision training, 160–161
  plus- and minus-to-blur findings,
    21–22
  proximal convergence, 28–29
  stimulus ACA ratio, 13
  strabismus, 177–179
  test results, 175–176
  vergence, 41
  zone of clear single binocular vision,
    23, 24–28, 34
Griffin, J. R., 175
Grisham, J. D., 95, 174–175

Hall, P., 140
Hart charts, 157, 217
Haynes, H. M., 137
Hofstetter, H., 2, 36, 47, 121, 141
Hogan, R. E., 174

Jackson, T. W., 140

Lag of accommodation, 34–35,
    137–141
Lead of accommodation, 137, 141
Leibowitz, H. W., 174
Lenses, fixation disparity, 73–74; *See
    also* Prescriptions
Lens rock, 135–137, 217
Locke, L. C., 140
Low neutral dynamic retinoscopy,
    137, 139, 140

Maddox, E. E., 40
Maddox components of convergence,
    40–41, 171–172
Mallett, R. F. J., 80
Mallett far-point units, 76, 78
Mallett near-point units, 78–80, 217
MEM dynamic retinoscopy,
    137–138, 140
Meter angle, 173, 177
Minus-to-blur test, 6, 21–22, 25, 140
Monocular estimation method. *See*
    MEM dynamic retinoscopy
Monocular lens rock test, 137
Monocular lens rock vision training,
    156–157
Morgan, M., 62
Morgan's test norms and clinical
    analysis, 62–64
Motor fusion, 178

Narayan, B., 191
Near-point of accommodation (NPA),
    22–23
Near-point of convergence (NPC), 6,
    23, 95, 150–151
Near-point phoria, 11
Negative fusional convergence (NFC),
    41, 154–155
Negative fusional reserve convergence
    (NFRC), 41, 47
Negative relative accommodation
    (NRA), 43–45, 140
Negative relative convergence (NRC),
    41, 47, 97
NFC. *See* Negative fusional convergence
NFRC. *See* Negative fusional reserve
    convergence

Night myopia, 174
Normal retinal correspondence, 179
Normative analysis, 63
Nott, I. S., 139
NPA. *See* Near-point of accommodation
NPC. *See* Near-point of convergence
NRA. *See* Negative relative accommodation
NRC. *See* Negative relative convergence

OEP. *See* Optometric Extension Program
One-to-one rule, 51–52
Optical reflex accommodation, 173, 174
Optometric Extension Program (OEP), 185–188
Orthophoria, 14
Orthoptic vision training. *See* Vision training
Owens, D. A., 174

Paradoxical fixation disparity, 70
Paralysis of accommodation, 142
Parasympatholytic drugs, 172
Parasympathomimetic drugs, 172
Payne, C. R., 107
PCT ratio, 171, 173
Percival's criterion, 53–56
PFC. *See* Positive fusional convergence
PFRC. *See* Positive fusional reserve convergence
Phoria line, 25, 165, 176, 188–190
Phorias
    associated phoria, 70, 71, 109
    basic esophoria, 103–105, 108
    basic exophoria, 101–103, 108
    dissociated phoria, 6, 9, 69, 70, 71, 76, 195
    distance phoria, 11
    esophoria, 42, 43, 47, 50–51, 76, 85
    exophoria, 9, 12, 42, 43, 47–50, 76, 85, 101–105, 125
    graphical analysis, 9–15, 176
    measurement, 76–81, 109
    near-point phoria, 11
    orthophoria, 14
    uncompensated phoria, 80, 82
    vertical phoria, 195–197
Phoria test, 41
Plus lenses, fixation disparity, 74

Plus-to-blur test, 6, 21–22, 25, 140
Positive fusional convergence (PFC), 41
    fixation disparity, 69
    vision training, 150–151, 154–155
Positive fusional reserve convergence (PFRC), 41, 47
Positive relative accommodation (PRA), 43–45, 97, 140
Positive relative convergence (PRC), 41, 47, 95
PRA. *See* Positive relative accommodation
Pratt system, 188–190
PRC. *See* Positive relative convergence
Presbyopia, 120–129
Prescriptions
    from associated phorias, 80, 82, 109
    from fixation disparity curves, 84–87
    graphical analysis, correlation, 176
    nonpresbyopic accommodative disorders, 141–146
    OEP analysis, 185–188
    using Percival's criterion, 53–56
    presbyopia, 121–123, 125–129
    prism adaptation, 71, 171, 191
    prism correction, 47, 51, 71, 85–86, 99, 107, 109, 185, 195–196
    using Sheard's criterions, 47–52
    vergence disorders, 41–45, 94–107
    vertical imbalance, 195–196
Prism adaptation, 71, 170–171, 191
Prism correction
    divergence insufficiency, 99
    fixation disparity, 85–86
    OEP analysis, 185
    Sheard's criterion, 47, 51
    studies, 107, 109
    vergence adaptation, 71
    vertical imbalance, 195–196
Prism diopter, 2, 4
Prism flippers, 175
Prism rock, 159
Proximal accommodation, 173
Proximal convergence, 11, 28–29, 35–38, 40, 171
Pseudoconvergence insufficiency, 35, 94, 105–108
Psychic convergence, 40

Push-up test, 120, 136
Push-up training, 150–151

Reduced fusional vergence, 105, 108
Response ACA ratio, 34
Retinoscopy
  dark focus, 174
  dynamic, 137–139, 140, 217
Rosenfield, M., 173
Rouse, M. W., 136, 138
Rutstein, R. P., 196

Saladin, J. J., 47, 51, 76, 84
Scheiman, M., 196
Schor, C. M., 76, 84, 169, 171, 191
Sheard's criterion, 34, 47–52, 76,
    100–101, 160
Sheedy, J. E., 47, 51, 68, 76, 82,
    84, 125
SILO response, 173
Slow fusional vergence, 171
Somers, W., 140
Spectacle plane, 177
Stimulus ACA ratio, 12–13, 35
Stimulus to accommodation, 2–6
Strabismus, 177–179
Suppression, 178

Tonic convergence, 11, 40
Tranaglyphs, 154, 217
Triad convergence, 168
Tropia line, 177–178

Uncompensated phorias, 80, 82

Vectograms, 154–155, 217
Vectographic slide, 76–77, 79, 80, 217
Vergence
  demand on vergence, 191–192
  Percival's criterion, 54
  types, 40–45
Vergence adaptation, 71, 171

Vergence disorders
  prescriptions, 41–45, 94–112
  vision training, 95, 97–99, 101, 102,
    106–107
Vergence facility, 174–175
Vertical fixation disparity, 196
Vertical fusional amplitude, 195–196
Vertical imbalances, 195–197
Vision training
  accommodative disorders, 141,
    150–161, 191
  binocular lens rock, 156
  Brock string, 152–153
  chiastopic fusion targets, 159–160
  convergence disorders, 150–161, 191
  distance rock, 157–158
  equipment sources, 217
  graphical analysis to plan, 160–161
  monocular lens rock, 156–157
  Percival's criterion, 54, 56
  prism rock, 159
  push-up training, 150–151
  Sheard's criterion, 47, 48, 51
  tranaglyphs, 154
  vectograms, 154–155
  vergence disorders, 95, 97–99, 101,
    102, 106–107
  vertical imbalance, 196
von Graefe prism dissociation tech-
    nique, 109

Wick, B., 84, 140, 196

Zone of clear single binocular vision
    (ZCSBV)
  accommodation and convervence,
    164–167
  depth of focus, 170
  graphical analysis, 23, 24–28, 34,
    140, 176
  Percival's criterion, 53–54
  presbyopia, 124–125